NATURALLY GORGEOUS

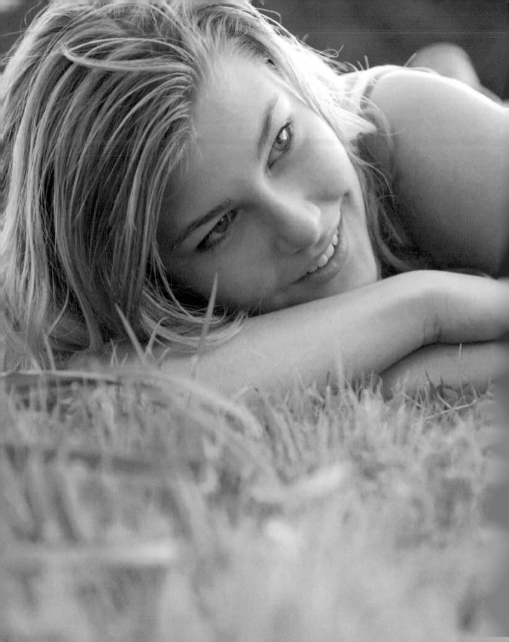

NATURALLY GORGEOUS

GORGEOUS

Essential Health and Beauty Secrets

Charlotte Vøhtz

EBURY
PRESS

" To my wonderful family, devoted staff and
all seekers of optimum health and natural beauty "

10 9 8 7 6 5 4 3 2 1

Published in 2007 by Ebury Press,
an imprint of Ebury Publishing
A Random House Group Company

The Random House Group Limited
Reg. No. 954009

Addresses for companies within the
Random House Group can be found at
www.randomhouse.co.uk

A CIP catalogue record for this book is
available from the British Library.

The Random House Group Limited makes
every effort to ensure that the papers used in
our books are made from trees that have been
legally sourced from well-managed and credibly
certified forests. Our paper procurement policy
can be found on www.randomhouse.co.uk

To buy books by your favourite authors and
register for offers visit www.rbooks.co.uk

Printed and bound in China by C & C Offset

ISBN 9780091922528

Text © Charlotte Vøhtz 2007
Illustrations © Liane Payne
Photographs © Green People
(models: Sandra Vøhtz Petersen,
Emily Sheldrake, Kendall Bradford),
except the following pages: Digital Vision: 41;
Getty Images: 25, 29, 74, 91, 106, 111, 128,
157, 168, 197; iStockphoto: 103, 107;
Stockbyte: 55, 94, 114, 133, 143, 205.

Designer: Isobel Gillan
Project editor: Anne McDowall
Copy editor: Richard Emerson

contents

praise for green people

"Charlotte is a true beauty pioneer – she believed in organic living long, long before it was fashionable, and I've always been inspired by her principles – and also by her wonderful products, which are proof that it's possible to be ethical and glamorous, all at the same time!"

JOSEPHINE FAIRLEY, JOURNALIST AND BEAUTY EDITOR

"Charlotte's vision for Green People is to make its already excellent service yet more bespoke, as this will give companies founded on ecological principles the edge in the future."

KATE SHAPLAND, JOURNALIST AND BEAUTY EDITOR OF THE *TELEGRAPH*

"I like to be low maintenance with my beauty routine and I try and use the purest products ... I like Green People products as they make the most gentle creams for the face and body, and their holistic approach works."

DARYL HANNAH, ACTRESS

"I always use Green People's sunscreens as they don't irritate my skin, are fabulous to use, highly effective and I trust their ingredients."

HAZEL COURTENEY, ALTERNATIVE HEALTH AUTHOR

"I confess it didn't even occur to me to think about what I was putting on my body until I had my first baby nine years ago. Confronted with that precious baby skin I realised I really did need to look for organic natural skincare and finding out about Green People was wonderful. I love the whole range and use their face oils, cleansers, and have even converted my hubby to the 'male grooming' products. My kids love the mandarin toothpaste and we are never without the organic sun block. A totally ethical company committed to natural products."

JANEY LEE GRACE, RADIO AND TV PRESENTER, AND AUTHOR

"Modern life is so toxic, so I avoid chemicals. I like Green People Aloe Vera Shampoo & Conditioner."

GABBY LOGAN, TV PRESENTER

introduction

I believe that we should all know the secrets of achieving radiant, natural beauty. After thirteen years of study and research into the field of organic health and beauty care I would now like to invite you to share in my best-kept beauty secrets.

My quest for an organic lifestyle began when my daughter Sandra, then aged two, developed eczema and skin allergies. Like every caring mother I wanted the best for her so was determined to find the cause of her health problems; the results of that search form the basis of this book.

Early on I came to realise that we are exposed to a chemical cocktail of hundreds of different compounds every day. Most of these chemicals are synthetic and man-made and did not exist until they were invented within the last few decades. This is a blink of the eye in evolutionary terms and our bodies just haven't learned how to deal with many of these chemicals.

Man-made chemicals are routinely found in our food, drinking water and the air we breathe; in the carpets, paints and furniture in our homes and workplaces; and in our clothes, household cleaners and personal care products. They are literally everywhere! This continuous exposure to chemicals places a great strain on the body's ability to cleanse and defend itself, and this can result in a build-up of toxins linked to many of the symptoms and chronic health problems that are so common these days.

Few of us are aware that products we use on a daily basis –
shampoos, shower baths, creams and lotions – are packed full of
man-made chemicals. I soon discovered that up to 60 per cent of
any chemical applied to the skin may be absorbed into the
bloodstream, adding further to the toxic burden. The need for
chemical-free personal care products for my daughter led me to
form The Green People Company and later became my impetus
to write this book.

My greatest reward is that more than ten years later, Sandra
(who is shown relaxing in the grass on page 2) and thousands of
others can enjoy good health and allergy-free skin by using natural
and organic skin care and avoid unnecessary synthetic chemicals.

The purpose of this book is to share my passion with you and
help you to avoid unnecessary man-made chemicals; and also to
suggest how you can cleanse your body of accumulated toxins,
both internally and externally.

I hope you enjoy reading *Naturally Gorgeous*, and that you will
find some of my tips useful towards achieving a greener lifestyle
and real organic beauty.

CHARLOTTE VØHTZ

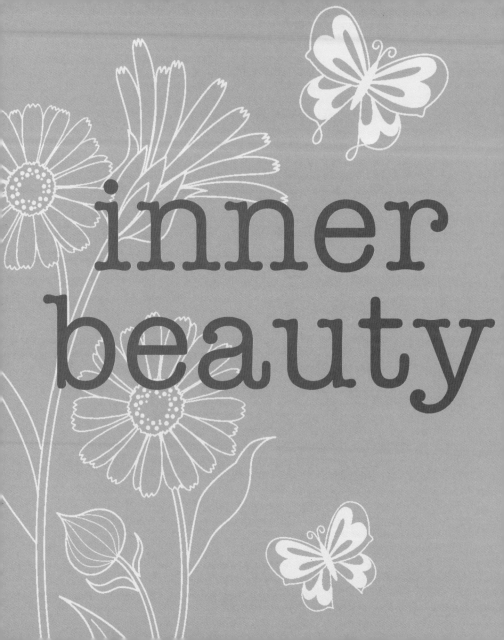

inner
beauty

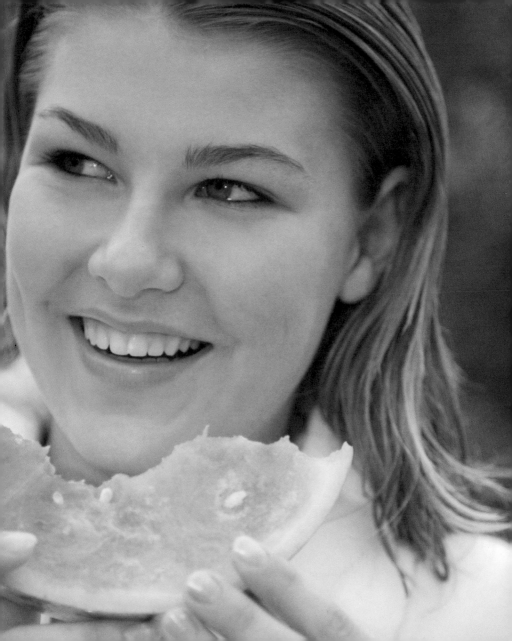

beauty from the inside out

Your skin is the body's largest organ and its condition is an indicator of your overall health. Healthy skin starts from within and proper nutrition is crucial to your looks and wellbeing. Eating a balanced nutrient-rich diet based on fresh organic produce, combined with moderate exercise and a positive outlook on life will all contribute to a glowing, radiant complexion.

If your skin is looking tired, sallow and prone to spots, you might wish to consider a detox (see pages 38–43). The health of your digestive system, your liver, the acidity of your blood and the way you breathe all affect your health and your looks. Drink plenty of fresh water throughout the day and increase your intake of dietary fibre and essential fatty acids.

● ●

INNER BEAUTY TIP **DON'T BE AFRAID OF FATS**

A clear complexion depends on a balanced, healthy diet rich in plenty of clean water, dietary fibre and essential fatty acids. Your skin cells are replaced every few days, so if you change how you eat, your skin will show signs of renewal after just a few weeks.

● ●

" Care for your digestive tract – it not only assists the removal of toxins but also releases vital energy for healing and elimination. "

absorbed directly into the blood stream

What you put on your skin can also affect your inner health. It is now known that up to 60 per cent of what comes into contact with the skin may be absorbed and can enter the bloodstream, from where it is transported to every organ of the body. Many ingredients used in mainstream cosmetics and personal care products are toxic to livings cells – examples include ethanol, synthetic perfumes and many preservatives. The same applies to household cleaning products, many of which contain potentially toxic ingredients.

emotional beauty

Inner peace is the foundation of outer beauty. Emotional beauty comes from a mind and heart that are in harmony. Happy, positive, loving individuals have a beauty that is far more than skin deep. Conversely we all experience the rapid and damaging effects on our skin from fatigue and stress. When mind and heart are at odds with each other it leads to emotional confusion, worry and loss of confidence, resulting in chronic stress.

Stress wrecks your health and plays havoc with your looks. It ages your face, makes your hair dull and your nails brittle, and puts strain and weight on your body. Raised stress-hormone levels narrow arteries and restrict blood flow. Your skin starts to look grey and lifeless. If you don't try to combat stress your skin will age prematurely.

INNER BEAUTY TIP **TRY REFLEXOLOGY**

As you enjoy a foot massage, you benefit from a better oxygen supply via the blood to all organs. Relaxation and relief of stress will immediately follow a reflexology session. Try it – your first reflexology session is unlikely to be your last!

" Shopping can lift your spirits. Give yourself a treat – go ahead and pamper yourself! "

tips to beat stress

Take time to beat stress – simple activities such as squeezing a stress ball or popping Bubble Wrap, thinking of your next holiday or having a giggle all help reduce stress. Here are some of my favourite stress busters:

* Take a five-minute break – go outside, flick through a magazine or have a power nap.
* Breathe slowly and deeply for a couple of minutes. Aim to do this several times a day.
* Eat a banana to boost your levels of the stress-busting hormone serotonin.
* Think of something funny. When you laugh you boost levels of endorphins ('feel-good' chemicals) in your body.
* Have a good stretch – raise your arms and stretch them over your head to relax a tense back and stiff shoulders.
* Hug a friend, cuddle your kids or kiss your partner.
* Focus your mind on a happy, memorable event in your life.

breathing

Your skin cells need plenty of oxygen to function properly. Without a ready supply of oxygen and efficient removal of carbon dioxide your skin won't feel smooth or have a healthy glow.

If you want beautiful skin you will also need plenty of fresh air. You should breathe in deeply to ensure the whole of the lungs are filled with oxygen-rich air, and then breathe out fully to expel as much of the stale, oxygen-depleted air as possible.

If your body doesn't get enough oxygen, you will start feeling tired, your complexion will become lacklustre and you will be more prone to thinning of the skin and premature wrinkling.

If your breathing is too shallow add more exercise to your daily routine and try deep-breathing exercises several times a day in the fresh air. Sleeping with the window open will help the air to circulate in your bedroom, filling your lungs with fresh air.

" Oxygen is essential to all living cells – deprived of this life-giving gas for just a few minutes, most of your body cells will starve and die. "

INNER BEAUTY TIP
TRY A ONE-MINUTE STRESS RELIEVER

If you feel stressed, put the tips of your fingers together, apply pressure and breathe slowly, counting to 60 while concentrating on your breathing.

bedtime breathing technique

If you are anxious or stressed your breathing is likely to be too fast. Try this simple exercise and notice the results immediately. You will feel your shoulders and arms relaxing, your chest will be less constricted and you will feel less stress and tension. Practise this technique every day until it becomes your natural routine, helping to induce natural sleep.

* Take a deep breath in through your nose and visualise the air moving down to your lungs. As you breathe in, silently count to four.
* Purse your lips as you exhale slowly through your mouth, silently counting to eight.
* Repeat this process eight to ten times.

the benefits of exercise

We all know how important it is to exercise, but did you know it also improves your skin? Exercise boosts blood flow throughout your body, increasing the supply of nutrients and oxygen and enhancing the removal of carbon dioxide and other acidic waste products. As a result your skin looks clearer and healthier and is less prone to premature ageing. Exercise also releases endorphins – natural 'feel-good' chemicals – so you will feel wonderful, too.

There are so many great ways to exercise – the choice is yours, but try to exercise outdoors in the fresh air. Brisk walking, cycling and weight-lifting improve cardiovascular fitness and muscular endurance, which translates into increased energy and a great complexion. Regular swimming builds endurance, muscle strength and cardiovascular fitness. It is also a great way to de-stress. Relax from the moment you take the first stroke, let your mind wander, focusing on nothing but the rhythm of your stroke.

incorporating exercise into your life

You don't have to join a gym to get fit: you can increase your fitness level simply by making the most of odd moments during the day to be active.

※ Pushing a lawn mower and raking leaves are all beneficial, low-impact ways to burn calories.

- ✳ Window cleaning is a good way to burn calories and work your upper body.
- ✳ Walk up a flight of stairs, and then back down (even at a slow pace) for just 5–10 minutes for a simple yet effective workout.
- ✳ Do standing wall pushes while you wait for the kettle to boil.
- ✳ Watching TV is no excuse! During the commercial breaks, get down on the floor and alternate sit-ups and leg lifts. You'll be amazed at how many repetitions you can fit in during the commecials of a half hour programme.
- ✳ When watching your child or partner playing sport, walk around the field several times or pace back and forth. Any movement is better than just sitting or standing.
- ✳ Sign up for a charity fitness event, and get your family involved too. It will give you an incentive to exercise, and training for the event will help you meet your fitness objectives.

● ●

DID YOU KNOW? **REBOUNDING**

Rebounding is bouncing on a mini trampoline. According to NASA, it is ' the most efficient and effective exercise yet devised' . The aim is to perform a series of small, controlled movements. You do not need to bounce high or perform gymnastic tricks! And because it is zero-impact exercise, there is no strain on your joints. (For stockist see page 218.)

● ●

water: the elixir of life

Water is not only a life-sustaining drink, it also makes up more than half your body weight. Water is needed for every function your body performs. It carries vital elements, oxygen, hormones, enzymes and chemical messengers to all parts of the body, transports nutrients into the cells and keeps the cells hydrated. Drinking water

* rids the body of toxins
* maintains skin elasticity and suppleness and prevents dryness
* aids weight loss
* keeps body systems, including metabolism and digestion, functioning effectively
* gives you the energy (and hydration) necessary for exercise
* regulates your temperature through sweating
* helps you stay energised and alert
* prevents constipation
* cushions and lubricates joints and muscles

good sources of water

You do not need to just drink pure water to keep your body hydrated. You can also obtain plenty from water-rich fruits and vegetables. These also contain a mixture of natural nutrients and mineral salts (electrolytes) and are more easily absorbed by the body than pure water on its own.

what about coffee and tea?

Coffee, tea, and other caffeine-rich beverages can act as diuretics – increasing urine production – but you lose only a fraction of what you actually drink. One cup of coffee results in a net gain of about two-thirds of a cup of water. Regular caffeine consumers gain even more as regular exposure to the drug builds resistance to its diuretic effects. Although moderate consumption will not lead to excessive fluid loss, avoid getting your entire fluid intake from caffeine-rich beverages. If you enjoy a shot of espresso, copy the southern Europeans and drink it with a glass of water.

● ●

INNER BEAUTY TIP **WAKE UP TO LEMON WATER**

At night toxins rise to the surface and you need to flush them out. Start your day with a glass of pure lemon water: one part freshly squeezed lemon juice to nine parts water. You can drink this 15–20 minutes before a meal to speed up metabolism and aid digestion. Lemons are a rich source of vitamin C and other associated nutrients, and stimulate liver and kidney function to flush out toxins from the system.

● ●

are you getting enough water?

The average healthy person should pass urine four to eight times per day. A good sign of healthy kidneys is when your urine is a pale straw colour. Many health care professionals suggest drinking eight glasses of water, diluted juices or herbal teas each day, increasing this amount on hot days or when exercising. However, some experts say there is little scientific justification for this and suggest body weight may be a better guide. On this basis, a daily fluid intake of around 1/40th of your total body weight seems optimum. For example, someone weighing 70kg would need to drink around 1.75 litres per day to keep adequately hydrated.

when do you need extra water?

If you lack energy, feel constantly thirsty, and your urine is a dark amber colour you may not be drinking enough water. Older people, and pregnant or breastfeeding women may need to increase their fluid intake. You also need to consume extra

* in hot, humid weather
* in cold weather or at high altitudes
* after drinking alcohol
* when spending long periods of time in air-conditioned and/or centrally heated buildings
* before, during and after strenuous exercise

INNER BEAUTY TIP **DRINK WHILE EXERCISING**

Drink plenty of water before, during and after energetic exercise to maintain hydration levels and help reduce muscle cramping and premature fatigue. Diluted fruit juices are even better than plain water as they replace vital salts (electrolytes) as well.

Symptoms of moderate dehydration include:
* dry, wrinkled skin
* lack of skin elasticity
* dry lips, mouth and tongue
* cramping in the arms and legs
* sleepiness or irritability
* headaches
* tiredness
* digestive problems
* dark urine

● ●

INNER BEAUTY TIP **USE A WATER PURIFIER**

A home water purifier will maximise the health-giving properties of water.
There is a wide range available, from simple jug filters to whole-house
systems. Choose one that removes potentially harmful compounds such as
chlorine, bacteria and heavy metals, but leaves behind the beneficial trace
minerals that are essential to health.

● ●

drink or not with meals?

Never drink cold water with meals as it dilutes enzymes and acids
needed to digest food. If partially digested food enters the colon,
bacteria get to work on it, causing gas, microbial imbalances and,
over time, mucous plaque. Small amounts of alcohol can be
combined with a meal, so enjoy a glass of wine or two or add it to
your recipe. Enjoy a glass of fresh lemon water 15–20 minutes
before your meal to support digestion, or choose herbal tea or
plain warm water.

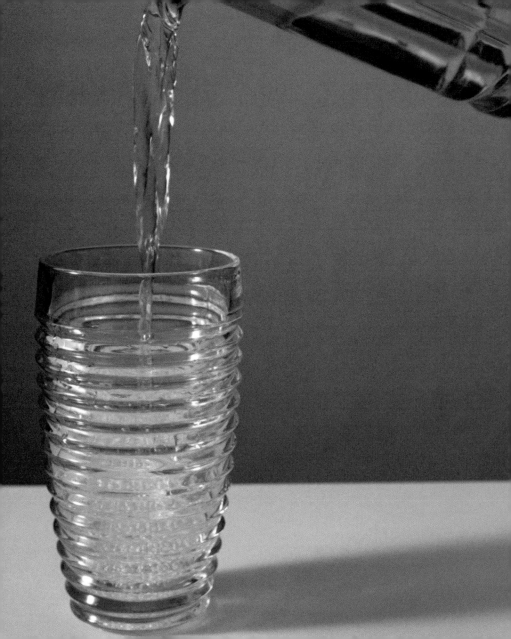

digestion

Nothing is more important to your overall health than the health of your digestive tract. Digestion begins in the mouth with the release of the enzyme salivary amylase, which breaks down starchy foods. To help the process, take small bites, chew thoroughly and put your fork down between mouthfuls. Avoid high-fat or calorie-dense meals just before bedtime. If you suffer poor digestion, avoid eating after 7pm.

Your capacity to make enzymes unfortunately diminishes with age and a chronic enzyme deficiency will result in poor digestion and inhibit your body from absorbing the nutrients it requires to sustain good health and radiant skin.

Poor habits such as inadequate chewing, and eating on the run, reduce enzyme production and lead to malabsorption of food. Avoid overeating and eat only when you are hungry. Regular exercise is a good way to build appetite and also provides your digestive tract with oxygenated blood.

● ●

INNER BEAUTY TIP **TRY KIMCHI**

Eat a little pickled, spicy food such as kimchi (pickled cabbage) or ginger before a meal to aid digestion.

● ●

relax when you eat

Stress and anger constrict the release of gastric juices so avoid eating when you feel angry or anxious. Don't eat while working at your computer, or when exercising or driving. Good digestion requires relaxation and enjoyment so do five minutes of deep breathing just before the meal. Practise mindful eating:

* Create a lovely atmosphere with fresh flowers and candlelight.
* Savour every bite, enjoying the flavours, textures and smells.
* Don't argue with your partner or kids at mealtimes – make the dining table a friction-free zone.

increase your fibre intake

A high-fibre diet helps your digestive tract function correctly. Good sources of fibre include fresh fruit; dried fruits, such as dates, figs, and prunes; vegetables; pulses (peas, beans and lentils) and nuts.

* Scandinavian-style crispbread (available in health food stores), made with 85 per cent unprocessed bran, is delicious with any topping and can replace regular bread in sandwiches or snacks.
* Supplement your diet with psyllium husks – remember to drink plenty of water when you increase your fibre intake.
* Ground flax seeds are a gentle laxative. Sprinkle some on rice, cereals, salads or any meal.

practice food combining

Protein needs different conditions for digestion from starchy foods, so avoid combining meat, eggs, cheese and fish with bread, rice, pasta, potatoes, yams and corn in the same meal. Proteins *or* carbohydrates can be combined with salads, and all vegetables, oils and nuts.

Enjoy breakfast cereals with rice or oat milk – and a banana if you like – but not cow's milk or soya milk, which don't mix well with starchy cereals.

Fruit is a 'superfood' able to pass quickly through your system, but avoid combining it with other foods as it interferes with protein and starch digestion. (You can eat fruit with yoghurt, as yoghurt is already partially digested. Live-culture yoghurt is an excellent source of beneficial bacteria, essential for a healthy colon and digestive system.) Ideally, eat fruit:

* first thing in the morning
* as a snack between meals
* when preparing an evening meal (but at least 15 minutes before the meal)

● ●

INNER BEAUTY TIP **GO EASY ON DESSERTS**

Don't eat carbohydrate-loaded desserts after a protein meal. Even fresh fruit eaten after a protein meal can cause havoc to your digestive system.

● ●

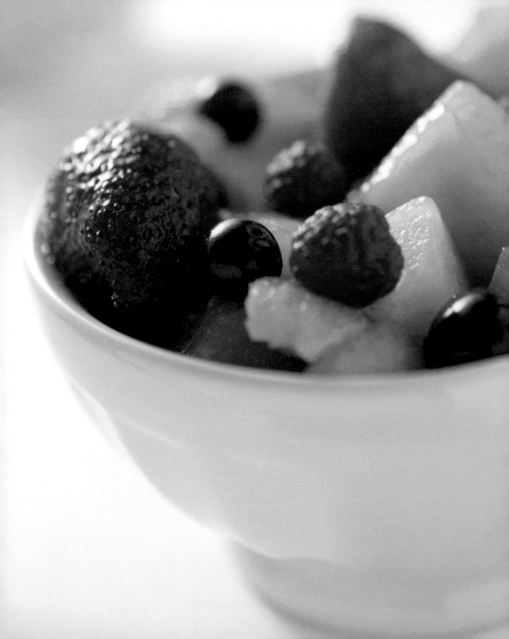

why eat organic?

Organic produce generally has a richer mineral content, due to a more balanced nutrient uptake in the absence of artificial fertilisers. It is not only the mineral content that is higher; organic foods are packed with vitamins and antioxidants, too. For example, milk from organically reared cows, fed on a diet of fresh grass, clover pasture and grass clover silage, has not only more antioxidants but also higher levels of omega-3 essential fatty acids. On average, compared with non-organic milk, it is:

* 50 per cent higher in vitamin E (alpha tocopherol)
* 75 per cent higher in beta carotene (precursor of vitamin A)
* 200–300 per cent higher in antioxidants lutein and zeaxanthin.

" Organic farming is better for wildlife, causes less pollution from sprays and produces less carbon dioxide and less dangerous wastes. "

the perils of pesticides

Conventionally grown fruit and vegetables can receive up to 20 chemical treatments, some of which are sprayed directly onto the skin, where 10–25 per cent of the residues may be absorbed into the flesh. Children are at greatest risk from pesticides as they eat more food, relative to body mass, especially juices, fresh fruits and vegetables, which are higher in pesticide residues.

Organic food is grown without the routine use of chemicals. Even after thorough washing, many fruits and vegetables consistently carry much higher levels of pesticide residue than organically grown. There are certain foods you should always buy organic, because of the potential threat from pesticide residues, especially in non-organic imported fruits. They include: apples, carrots, celery, cherries, grapes, lettuce, nectarines, peaches, pears, peppers, potatoes, raspberries, rice, spinach, strawberries, sunflower seeds and tomatoes.

DID YOU KNOW? **PESTICIDES AND GROWTH**

Exposure to low levels of pesticides at crucial stages in foetal and infant development can damage or disrupt human hormonal, neurological, reproductive and immune systems.

do you pass the acid test?

Cells live in an almost neutral environment – neither too acidic nor too alkaline. A good diet containing mainly alkaline-producing foods maintains this healthy cellular environment. However, the typical Western diet is too high in acid-producing products such as red meat, eggs and sugar-rich foods, and far too low in alkaline-producing foods such as fresh vegetables.

Additionally, most of the population eat too much acid-producing processed foods such as white flour and sugar, and drink acid-producing beverages such as coffee and soft drinks. Artificial chemical sweeteners such as aspartame, acesulfame K and saccharin are especially acid forming.

Holistic therapists and nutritionists consider a properly balanced diet to be important to optimal health and in preventing diseases such as arthritis, heart disease and even cancer.

the problem of acidity

Normal healthy blood is slightly alkaline. Acidic blood will harm the cells' ability to

* absorb minerals and other nutrients
* generate energy
* repair damage
* remove toxins

In addition to an acid-producing diet, excess acidity can also be caused by

❊ emotional stress

❊ toxic overload

❊ immune reactions

❊ any process that deprives the cells of oxygen and other nutrients

Your body then has to correct the pH (see below) by utilising the body's store of alkaline minerals. When these reserves are depleted your body 'borrows' minerals from whatever source it can, usually the bones and vital organs. Over time this can lead to weaknesses in the skeleton and other affected organs.

● ●

DID YOU KNOW? **THE pH SCALE**

The pH scale runs from 1 to 14 and is a way of measuring the alkalinity or acidity of a substance, including blood and sweat. Water is neutral – neither acid nor alkaline – and is 7 on the pH scale. Anything below 7 is acid and anything above is alkaline (or a 'base'). The further the pH shifts from 7 – in either direction – the stronger (and potentially more irritating) it becomes. Healthy blood is slightly alkaline, around pH 7.35.

● ●

symptoms of excess acidity

There are various symptoms associated with excess acidity. Many of these are associated with other medical conditions, too, so seek qualified medical advice if they persist, especially after changing your diet to one with a more alkaline balance. Symptoms include:

* low energy, chronic fatigue
* excess mucus production
* nasal congestion
* frequent colds, flu and other infections
* feeling nervous, stressed, irritable, anxious, agitated
* weak nails, dry hair, dry skin
* headaches
* joint pain or arthritis
* neuritis
* muscle pain
* leg cramps and spasms
* gastritis, acid indigestion
* bladder and kidney problems
* weight gain

how to alkalinise your diet

A food's acid or alkaline-forming properties have little or nothing to do with the pH of the food itself. For example, lemons are very acidic but their end-products are very alkaline. Conversely, meat is alkaline but it leaves a very acidic residue in the body. To make your diet more alkaline:

- eat lots of fresh vegetables and fruit
- drink alkaline vegetable juices such as carrot, celery and beetroot
- drink green drinks – add barley grass powder to a glass of water or your smoothie
- drink plenty of water with a squeeze of lemon or lime
- drink herbal teas instead of coffee and carbonated soft drinks
- eat at least one serving daily of greens, such as green beans, cabbage or broccoli
- cut out white bread, white pasta and white rice completely
- use flax oil or omega-3 and -6 blends in your salad dressing and use organic virgin olive oil for cooking

DID YOU KNOW? **DIGESTIVE ENZYMES**

As we get older we may not produce sufficient digestive enzymes and so partially digested food can enter the intestines or remain longer in the stomach, becoming more acidic. Enzyme supplementation helps treat this problem. Look for supplements containing a range of enzymes, including pepsin, lipase, amylase and protease as these help to digest a wide range of different food types.

strongly acid forming foods

beef, crab meat, eggs (whole), herring, lamb, liver, lobster, mackerel, organ meats, pork, prawns, biscuits, cakes, couscous, white bread, white rice, white pasta, yeasted breads, beer, wine, spirits, black tea, carbonated water, hot chocolate, coffee, fizzy drinks, readymade lemonade, artificial sweeteners, hydrogenated fats, lard and suet, margarine, mayonnaise, molasses, mushrooms, mustard, processed foods, tinned foods, white sugar

mildly acid forming foods

sea bass, cheese, chicken, cream, egg yolks, halibut, lemon sole, milk (UHT), mussels, oysters, salmon, trout, tuna, turkey, yoghurt (sweetened), apples, apricots, blueberries, grapes, kiwi fruit, melons (except watermelon), oranges, mandarins, peaches, pears, pineapple, plums, raspberries, redcurrants, strawberries, brown rice, millet, oats, quinoa, rye, spelt, wholegrain cereals, wholegrain pasta, fructose, honey, malt vinegar, maple syrup, pickles, sugar (raw cane), wine vinegar

mildly alkaline forming foods

brie and camembert cheese (young), milk (pasteurised), yoghurt (fresh, plain), artichoke, buckwheat, cauliflower, lentils, mung beans, onions, garden peas, red kidney beans, tofu, apple cider vinegar, green tea, herbs (fresh or dried), lemonade (fresh, low sugar), mineral water (non-carbonated), mint tea, sea salt, soya milk (unsweetened), tomato juice, vegetable juices (fresh), vegetable oils (cold pressed only)

strongly alkaline forming foods

peppers, beetroot, broccoli, Brussels sprouts, butter beans, carrots, celery, courgettes, cucumber, garlic, grains (e.g. barley, wheat), green beans, cabbage, leeks, peas, potatoes, radishes, salad greens, soya beans, spinach, sweetcorn, turnips, watercress, avocadoes, bananas, cherries, coconut, grapefruit, lemons, limes, watermelon

test your pH level

The easiest way to monitor your progress on the alkaline diet is to check the pH of your urine using pH test strips available from your local pharmacy (or see page 218 for stockists).

Urine provides a fairly accurate picture of true body chemistry, because the kidneys filter out the salts used to balance pH. Urine pH can vary from 4.5 to 9.0, with the ideal range being around 6.0 to 7.0.

● ●

INNER BEAUTY TIP **CALCIUM AND MAGNESIUM**

If your urine test shows a lower pH value than the optimums given above, you may benefit from supplementing your diet with calcium and magnesium. Supplement with vitamins A and D to help hold calcium in the body. Take psyllium husk in plenty of water at bedtime to maintain regular bowel movements.

● ●

getting the balance right

To restore health if your system is too acidic, your diet should contain 80 per cent alkaline-forming foods and 20 per cent acid-forming foods. Then, to maintain good health, your diet should consist of around 60 per cent alkaline-forming foods and 40 per cent acid-forming foods.

detoxify your body

Synthetic chemicals are everywhere – in the air, food, drinking water and all around us in the home. Cigarette smoke, alcohol, junk food, medicines and personal care products all add to this toxic overload. Nearly every cell in the body has the ability to break down toxins. But those in the liver carry out the lion's share of this activity. How well the liver performs this complicated job depends on your genes and the extent of the chemical burden you are under. Detoxification also occurs in the gut lining. Factors such as bacterial balance and the presence of food additives, pesticides and preservatives can all have an adverse effect.

A great way to improve your health and boost your wellbeing is to cleanse your body of its accumulated toxins by following a detoxification programme. You'll be surprised how great it makes you look and feel. Detox can take from one day up to several weeks. If it is your first time, 2–3 days will make a big difference.

" The safest place for excess toxins to overflow is through the skin because this is the furthest away from vital organs. Spots and pimples can be the result of toxins being eliminated through your skin. "

side effects of detox

Detoxing can cause a strong physical as well as mental reaction. As toxins work their way out of your tissues into the bloodstream you will probably experience side effects. Common symptoms include spots, rashes, headaches, body odour, bad breath, nausea and a runny nose, diarrhoea or constipation. You may experience flu-like symptoms, slight depression or mood swings. Avoid painkillers, and drink plenty of filtered or bottled water with a twist of lemon.

● ●

INNER BEAUTY TIP **SPEED UP YOUR DETOX**

The detox process will work more efficiently if you eat organic produce. Choose fruits and vegetables with powerful detox properties such as apples, grapes, kiwi fruit, lemon, pears, strawberries, artichoke, beetroot, broccoli, cabbage, carrots, celery, lettuce, nettle, onion and watercress.

● ●

detox supplements

The following supplements aid the detox process and/or supply additional nutrients your body needs.

✳ Soluble fibre mixes with water to form a gel. It soothes the digestive tract, prevents constipation and helps remove toxins. Good sources include psyllium husks and cracked flax seeds. Always drink plenty of water when taking extra fibre.

❉ Edible clay traps toxins and carries them out of the body. Be sure to buy food-grade clay and follow the instructions supplied. Good examples include Montmorillonite and Bentonite. Drink plenty of water. Clay can be combined with soluble fibre, too.

❉ Wild seaweed (kelp) supplies essential minerals, vitamins and trace elements in natural balance. It also has cleansing and diuretic properties that aid the detox process.

❉ Other nutrient-rich supplements include spirulina or chlorella, both single-celled plants, which can be taken as tablets, capsules or as a powder, mixed into water or diluted juices.

❉ The herb milk thistle offers excellent support for your liver.

❉ Ginger helps support your digestive system.

● ●

INNER BEAUTY TIP **FOLLOW MEDICAL ADVICE**

If you have any health problems consult your health practitioner before attempting a detox. If you are pregnant, do not follow a detox diet but enrich your diet with plenty of fruits and vegetables, herbal teas and water and avoid coffee and alcohol.

● ●

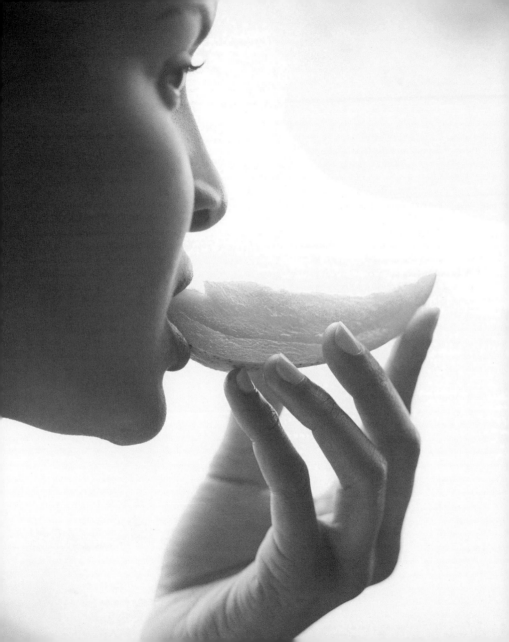

the detox diet programme

Plan your detox diet well ahead. The week before hide any
tempting processed, fatty and sugary foods; cut out tea,
coffee, sugar, bread, meat, alcohol and tobacco (and continue to
avoid them for a few days after the detox has ended). Drink lots of
fresh water and introduce more organic fruit, vegetables and
juices and eat lots of brown rice and steamed vegetables. Prepare
your system by taking a spoonful of psyllium husk or linseeds with
a large glass of water.

day one

* **Morning:** Drink a glass of cooled boiled water with the juice
of half a lemon.
* **Throughout the day:** Eat grapes whenever you feel hungry.
Aim to eat at least 1kg during the day. Drink plenty of filtered
or bottled water, herbal teas (try peppermint, chamomile, ginger
or Yogi Teas) and freshly squeezed, carrot, celery and apple
juice. Dilute all juices 50:50 with filtered or bottled water. Aim
to drink a minimum of eight glasses (200ml each) of liquid a
day, with no more than half of this being diluted juices – the
rest should be water or non-diuretic herbal teas.

day two

❊ **Morning:** Drink a glass of cooled boiled water with the juice
of half a lemon.

❊ **Throughout the day:** Drink filtered or bottled water, herbal
teas and vegetable juice made from any of the organic
vegetables listed on page 39. Again, dilute with water: one part
vegetable juice to one part water, and aim for a minimum eight
glasses of liquid during the day, at least half of which should be
water or herbal teas (see also pages 46–7).

day three

❊ **Morning:** Eat raw fruits from the list on page 39. Eat as much
as you like. Drink plenty of filtered or bottled water and herbal
teas. If you don't like eating raw fruit, create fresh juice blends.

❊ **Lunch:** Vegetable medley made with organic vegetables from
the list on page 39 – raw or steamed, as you prefer. Drink
plenty of filtered or bottled water and herbal teas.

❊ **Supper:** Soup made with vegetables from the list on page 39.
Drink plenty of filtered or bottled water and herbal teas.

after your detox

Re-introduce coffee, alcohol, sugar, bread, meats and so on slowly
– and only at all if you can't live without them. Support the inner
cleansing process with a gentle daily detox drink based on enzyme-
rich plant juices, such as Hawthorn & Artichoke Formula (see
page 218). The detox diet can be repeated every three months.

plant foods for your skin

Skin health depends on following a diet rich in high-quality nutrients. If you want beautiful skin you must limit or avoid processed foods, sugar, saturated fat, cigarette smoke, excess sunlight and alcohol, all of which increase free radical production.

antioxidants – skin defenders

Antioxidants fight free radicals. They restore skin health, promote healing and combat premature skin ageing. Antioxidants are also the most powerful natural defence against cancer. Many fruits and vegetables contain compounds with antioxidant properties.

As well as vitamins and minerals, these include phytonutrients (plant nutrients), such as lutein, found in tomatoes; quercetin, found in many dark coloured berries and red wine; and hesperidin, found in citrus fruits. Rich sources of antioxidants include

* fruits: blueberries, blackberries, raspberries, grapes, oranges and kiwi
* vegetables: kale, spinach, broccoli, beetroot, Brussels sprouts and onions are equally rich sources

● ●

DID YOU KNOW? **FREE RADICALS**

Free radicals are highly reactive molecules that destroy cells and tissues, leading to premature ageing and decay. They attack the moist collagen fibres that give the skin elasticity, leading to a dry, wrinkled appearance.

● ●

the skin's miracle workers

Plant chemicals called flavonoids and isoflavones can also slow signs of ageing and restore your beauty. These plant pigments help foster a healthy blood supply to the skin by strengthening tiny blood vessels. They work in conjunction with vitamin C.

Flavonoids protect your skin from ageing, premature wrinkles and skin damage caused by UV light. Flavonoids help alleviate fluid retention, allergies, haemorrhage, heavy menstrual bleeding and high blood pressure. They are found in green tea, apples, cranberries, celery, onions, kale, parsley, beetroot, soya beans and tomatoes.

Isoflavones not only act as antioxidants but also have weak hormone-like properties that aid health problems associated with hormone imbalances such as PMS, menopausal symptoms and breast cancer. They are present in beans (especially soya beans), wholegrains, fruits (especially berries) and brightly coloured vegetables.

carotenoids

There are 500 or more carotenoids in food plants, especially dark green and orange ones like kale, broccoli, spinach, yellow squashes, peppers, carrots and apricots. Research shows carotenoid levels in tissues are also critical in determining life span. Skin that is dry, rough, scaly, or pimpled will benefit from carotenes. A 454ml glass of carrot juice not only contains 5g of protein, and a respectable 35mg of vitamin C but also 100,000 IU of betacarotene, a water-soluble carotenoid that the body converts into vitamin A as needed.

" A home-made smoothie rich in organic fresh fruit and blended with barley grass and omega oils is my favourite way of starting the day. "

fresh juices – 'live' enzymes

Adding fresh juices to your diet will boost the nutrient value of your diet and help make your skin glow. There's no better way to obtain all the nutrients you need than by consuming live (uncooked) plant foods and fresh juice. They're great for meeting everyday energy demands, and taken with meals they help digest other food.

By reducing the amount of work your body must perform for digestion, you liberate extra energy for the cells and everything they do. Live juices conserve your internal enzyme supply whereas cooked foods don't have any enzymes and therefore deplete your own supplies.

Nutrients from juices are assimilated in minutes for instant energy and cell regeneration. Made with or without pulp in juicers and blenders, they provide a concentrated source of live enzymes, minerals, vitamins, antioxidants, flavonoids, carotenoids and other phytonutrients.

INNER BEAUTY TIP **BEWARE HEAT-TREATMENT**

Most so-called 'fresh juices' are pasteurised to extend their shelf-life. Heat treatment not only kills the bacteria that cause food spoilage but also destroys the enzymes present naturally in the raw plant. The answer is to make your own juices and drink them while still fresh.

sprouting

Sprouted seeds offer a superb source of skin-essential nutrients. Sprouting improves the nutritional value of all seeds and makes them more easily digestible. Sprouts contain an abundance of highly active antioxidants that prevent DNA destruction and help protect you from premature ageing. They preserve the health of the skin, by aiding healing and rejuvenation processes, and enhance its glow.

Regular use of sprouted products helps to maintain the internal purity of the system, reducing the risk of long-term skin eruptions, acne or other skin disorders. For their food value, there is nothing to beat them. Make them a regular part of your diet.

what can I sprout?

Sprouting needs little effort. Most seeds, grains and pulses can be sprouted, including wheat, millet, maize, fenugreek seeds, coriander seeds, sunflower seeds, alfalfa, radish, broccoli, clover, lentils, chickpeas and soya beans – the list is endless. Even better, they can be grown anywhere. You don't need purpose-made sprouting trays, the easiest and cheapest way is to use glass jars. Encourage your kids to sprout, they'll love it!

how to sprout

* Use a clean, clear glass jar (such as a large jam jar). Add one or two teaspoons of your chosen seeds and half-fill the jar with cold water. Stretch a piece of thin cloth (muslin is ideal) over the neck and secure with an elastic band.

* Leave to soak for a few hours – or overnight for larger seeds, such as soya beans and chick peas.

* Pour the water away through the muslin cover and place in a warm position (about 20°C) with natural light, but out of direct sunlight.

* Twice a day, rinse the seeds in cold water, draining thoroughly. Turn the jar each time you rinse so the seeds get an equal amount of light and grow evenly. Your sprouts will be ready to eat after four or five days.

* Place in sealed bags, so that they stay flavourful and crisp. If necessary, rinse in cold water daily. Rinse the sprouts thoroughly before eating, and store the excess in the refrigerator for two to three days.

* Add sprouts to your meals to boost your intake of skin nutrients.

essential fats

Many people believe the key to good health is to 'cut out all fats'. But fats are not created equal. Some increase your risk of disease but others promote health. So cutting out all fats is not a good idea. The ones to avoid are the saturated fats. They are found primarily in meat, dairy products and processed foods. Saturated fats offer little nutritional benefit and when eaten in excess can cause health problems including raised cholesterol and heart disease. In addition, excess consumption of saturates increases the risk of blocked, infected pores.

The key to good health is to replace bad fats with good fats. 'Good' fats are unsaturated – mono-unsaturated and polyunsaturated – and have many health benefits. They help the body absorb nutrients, aid nerve transmission, maintain cell membranes, and much more.

mono-unsaturated fats

The richest source of mono-unsaturated fatty acids is olive oil, which helps to prevent the creation and accumulation of harmful cholesterol in the body. People who follow a Mediterranean diet, which is based on olive oil, have relatively low levels of cholesterol with correspondingly little incidence of heart disease. Other rich sources of mono-unsaturated fatty acids include rapeseed oil, nuts and peanut butter.

polyunsaturated fats

Polyunsaturated fatty acids (PUFAs) have many important functions in the body. Some – called essential fatty acids (EFAs) – are vital for the health of the nerves, heart and circulation and are used to make hormone-like substances that control many other body systems. They are called 'essential' because they must be obtained from the diet – the body can't make them. EFAs enhance absorption of vitamins and minerals and nourish hair, skin and nails. EFAs fall into two groups: omega-6 and omega-3.

Omega-6 fatty acids include linoleic acid and gamma-linolenic acid and are abundant in evening primrose oil, borage oil and blackcurrant seed oil. Many experts recommend taking omega-6 with omega-3 fatty acids for their synergistic effect.

Omega-3 fatty acids are often lacking in the Western diet. Key omega-3 fatty acids include eicosapentaenoic acid (EPA) and docosahexanoic acid (DHA). They are primarily found in coldwater oily fish such as salmon, tuna and mackerel. A third type, alpha-linolenic acid (ALA), is found in plant-derived foods such as dark green, leafy vegetables and flax seed oil.

"If you want softer skin, get plenty of omega fatty acids in your diet. Not only do they improve your skin but you will also have more energy, improved concentration and will feel happier and less stressed."

benefits of EFAs

Dry, flaky skin, dull hair, dandruff and brittle nails are often a result of an imbalance of EFAs. Your skin cells need plenty of 'good' fat. Internally administered, the right balance of omega-3 and omega-6 has been shown to

* moisturise the skin from the inside, making it softer, smoother and healthier and helping to prevent dry skin and other conditions including eczema, psoriasis, and atopic dermatitis
* have an anti-inflammatory effect on the skin
* boost concentration and learning, especially in children
* help alleviate premenstrual and menopausal symptoms and reduce mood swings
* be necessary for hormone production

taking omega-3 and -6 oils

There are several good plant-based blends on the market. Choose one rich in flax seed oil – especially if you don't eat fish.

※ Take 1–2 tablespoons daily on vegetables, blended in a 'health cocktail' or in a salad dressing.

※ Essential fatty acids spoil easily. Do not use for cooking, and once opened keep refrigerated.

※ To be most effective, combine with protein at the same meal.

※ For optimum results, reduce stress and eliminate substances that promote it such as refined sugar, soda, coffee and fluoride.

● ●

DID YOU KNOW? **FLAX SEED OIL**

Flax seed oil not only provides an average of 58 per cent omega-3 and 14 percent omega-6, but it is also rich in beta carotene and vitamin E. The Cherokee Indians prized it highly, believing it captured the sun's energy.

● ●

skin vitamins and minerals

For really beautiful skin, you need to start from the inside. Making sure that your diet includes a good balance of vitamins and minerals will help minimise or prevent problems and enhance your skin's natural beauty.

vitamin A/beta carotene

Essential for healthy hair and eyes and to prevent and clear skin infections, vitamin A counteracts dry skin, dandruff and wrinkle formation and can help protect against sun damage. It is needed for healthy blood circulation, which gives a glow to your skin.

A deficiency can lead to eruptions or dry, wrinkled skin, dull and dry hair or dandruff, ridging or peeling fingernails, pimples or acne and visual fatigue.

vitamin B

Promoting clear, luminous skin and youthful looks, vitamin B is essential for healthy skin, hair and eyes. Studies show that 40 per cent of dermatitis sufferers lack B vitamins. B vitamins also help counteract stress, which has adverse effects on appearance.

A deficiency can lead to greasy hair, dandruff, dry skin, redness and irritation, premature wrinkles, poor hair growth, grey hair and inflamed fissures at the angles of the nose and mouth.

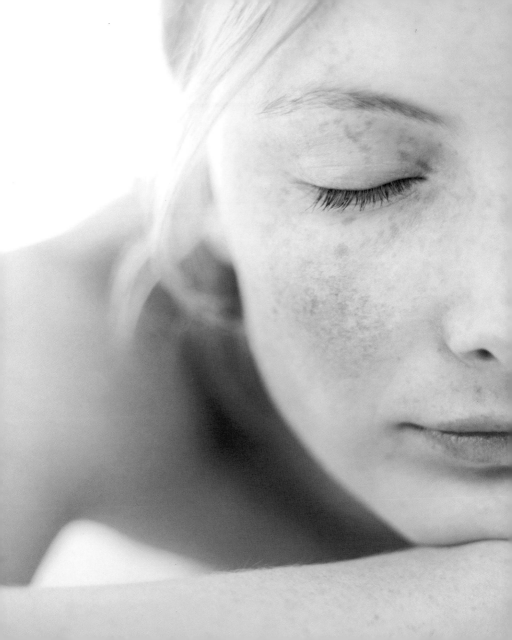

vitamin C

Vitamin C is necessary – in conjunction with protein – for the production of collagen, which is the 'glue' that holds us and our skin together and circumvents sags or wrinkles. It regulates sebaceous glands to keep skin from drying out and helps prevent facial lines, wrinkles and spider veins and hair tangling or breaking. Vitamin C is also essential for the health of the hair, eyes and teeth, resistance to infection, healing of wounds and firm skin tissues.

Combined with bioflavonoids, vitamin C prevents the pigment clumping that the sun turns into age spots, strengthens capillaries to avoid easy bruising or the tiny haemorrhages that become spider veins, helps the oil-secreting glands function properly to keep the skin from drying out and prevents bleeding of the gums.

vitamin D

Essential for healthy teeth, bones and nails as well as for the assimilation of calcium and phosphorus, vitamin D promotes healthy eyes, skin and teeth. A deficiency of vitamin D can lead to brittle bones and dental decay.

vitamin E

Helps form muscles and tissues to prevent wrinkles and premature skin ageing. It helps prevent dry, dull skin, age spots, hair loss and dandruff. It improves circulation and healing of scars. Warning: if you have diabetes, high blood pressure or an overactive thyroid, check with a health professional before taking supplemental E.

minerals

Minerals are just as important as vitamins in maintaining beautiful skin and are essential for all the body's activities. The lack of just one mineral can disturb this balance, leading to a wide range of possible health problems and symptoms.

* **Calcium and phosphorus** work together for healthy teeth, hair, nails and bones. Calcium helps clear blemished skin and revitalises lifeless, tired-looking skin.
* **Chromium** improves circulation for healthy skin and hair.
* **Copper** is important for the production of skin pigment and for the prevention of blotches under the skin from ruptured blood vessels. It also cooperates with other nutrients to preserve the integrity of the elastic-like fibres supporting the skin.
* **Iodine** promotes healthy hair, nails, skin and teeth.
* **Iron** is essential for healthy nails, skin colour and hair growth.
* **Magnesium** is required to prevent skin disorders.
* **Manganese** helps to maintain healthy hair.
* **Potassium** helps maintain healthy skin and prevent puffiness.
* **Selenium** maintains skin elasticity and helps prevent and correct dandruff. It helps safeguard the skin from sun damage.
* **Sulphur** helps maintain healthy hair, nails and skin. It also prevents dermatitis, eczema and psoriasis.
* **Zinc** helps prevent wrinkles, dry skin and stretch marks and promotes blemish healing. It prevents hair loss and brittle or spotted nails. Without enough zinc a deficiency of vitamin A can occur even though the intake of that vitamin is adequate.

natural sources of vitamins and minerals

Vitamins and minerals are found in a wide variety of foods and a balanced diet should provide you with the quantities you need.

vitamin A/beta carotene

Cod liver oil, liver, kidney, dairy, eggs, carrots, green leafy vegetables, tomatoes, papaya, pumpkin, melon, apricots, mangos

vitamin B complex

Brewer's yeast, green leafy vegetables, meat (especially liver), molasses, nuts, pulses, wholegrain cereals

vitamin C

Citrus fruits, cantaloupe melon, kiwi, strawberries, green vegetables, tomatoes, potatoes

vitamin D

Beef liver, dairy products, salmon, sprouted seeds, tuna. (Sunlight is also a source of vitamin D.)

vitamin E

Whole-wheat bread, whole grains, wheat germ, milk, raw or sprouted seeds, asparagus, broccoli, Brussels sprouts, butter, egg yolks, leafy greens, liver, olives, soya beans, sunflower seeds, nuts, vegetable oils

calcium and phosphorus

Dairy products, whole wheat, leafy vegetables, fish, poultry, meat, grains, cereals, soya beans, sunflower seeds, walnuts, fruit juices

chromium

Brewer's yeast, cheese, corn oil, liver, clams, meat, whole grains

copper

Beef and pork liver, chicken, leafy greens, mushrooms, nuts, raisins, shellfish (oysters), whole grains

iodine

Iodised salt, kelp, onions, seafood, vegetable oils

iron

Egg yolks, blackstrap molasses, dark leafy greens, dried fruits and legumes, lean meat, liver, whole wheat

magnesium

Almonds, apples, apricots, bananas, bran, corn, dairy products, figs, grapefruit, lemons, meat, raw leafy greens, soya beans

manganese

Bananas, bran, egg yolks, leafy greens, legumes, nuts and grains

potassium

Bananas, citrus and dried fruits, coffee, fresh vegetables, kiwi fruit, lean meats, legumes, peanuts, potatoes, tea

selenium

Asparagus, bran, broccoli, chicken, egg yolks, milk, onions, red meat, seafood, tomatoes, whole grains

sulphur

Bran, brussels sprouts, cabbage, cheese, clams, eggs, fish, mushrooms, nuts, peas and beans, wheat germ

zinc

Brewer's yeast, eggs, lean red meat, legumes, mushrooms, non-fat dry milk, pumpkin and sunflower seeds, shellfish (oysters), spinach, whole grains

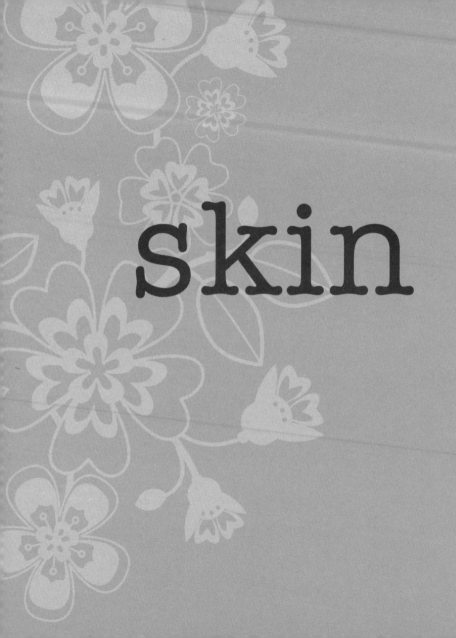

skin

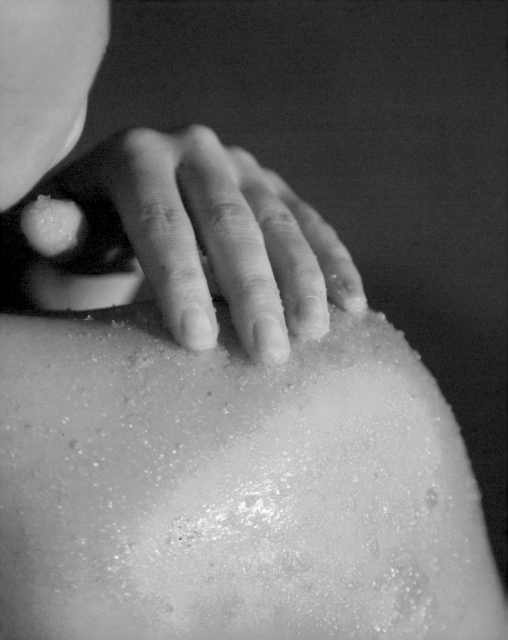

understanding your skin

Your skin is your first line of defence against dehydration, infection, injuries and extremes of temperature. It combines strength with elasticity to help resist knocks and shocks. The skin can be up to 5mm thick, but this varies over the body. The thickest areas are the palms and soles and the thinnest are the eyelids – just 0.3mm thick. Your skin is made up of layers – an upper layer or epidermis, and a lower layer or dermis. Below the dermis is the subcutaneous layer, containing fat and connective tissue, which shapes and cushions the body.

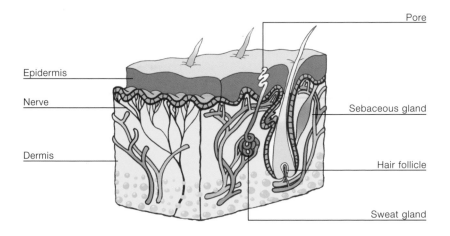

Pore

Epidermis

Nerve

Sebaceous gland

Dermis

Hair follicle

Sweat gland

the epidermis

The top layers of the epidermis are made up of dry, tightly knit cells filled with keratin, a fibrous protein (also found in hair and nails) that protects the skin and stops it drying out. These cells can absorb about five times their weight of water and swell to three times their original thickness.

The epidermis works ceaselessly to regenerate itself. The cells are born in the lowest layer of the epidermis and migrate upwards for about two weeks, during which time they flatten out and die. Eventually, the upper layer of dead cells is shed from the surface. Two to three billion skin cells are shed every day (they make up a substantial percentage of household dust).

The spaces between the epidermal cells are packed with natural fats (lipids). These fats help the top layer of dead skin cells regulate natural water loss. If they are removed by harsh soaps or detergents, or damaged by sunburn, the skin loses some of its ability to retain water and easily dries out.

the dermis

The base layer, the dermis, is mainly composed of a network of protein fibres: collagen and elastin. Collagen gives skin its strength and elastin keeps the skin supple and resilient. Collagen and elastin fibres are damaged by the effects of ageing, free radicals, pollutants, such as tobacco smoke, and UV light. By the age of 40, almost half the elastin present at birth is lost, resulting in lines, wrinkles and thin, sagging skin. The dermis houses the hair follicles, from which new hair is made, and sensory nerve receptors, responsible for the sense of touch, heat, cold and pain. It is also rich in tiny blood and lymph vessels to provide oxygen and nutrients for cell growth and repair and remove wastes.

sweat and oil glands

Within the dermis are the sweat and sebaceous glands, whose secretions reach the surface through tiny openings or pores. Sweat glands mainly regulate temperature.

Sebaceous glands produce an oily secretion called sebum, which lubricates and waterproofs the skin and helps prevent moisture loss. Sebaceous glands are most concentrated on the scalp and face – particularly around the nose, cheeks, chin and forehead, hence these are usually the oiliest areas. Sebum production can increase temporarily during stress, before your period and around the menopause. As we get older we tend to produce less sebum and the skin becomes drier.

the acid mantle

Skin and hair are protected by a thin sticky fluid, the acid mantle, formed from sebum, sweat, and acidic secretions produced by skin 'good' bacteria such as *Staphylococcus epidermis*. The acid mantle creates a hostile environment for 'bad' bacteria, which prefer an alkaline environment.

Any disruption to the acid mantle – e.g. excess sunlight, poor diet, alkaline skin products and harsh soap – interferes with the protective outer layer of the skin and strips away the acid mantle. This leads to dehydration, roughness and irritation. Skin is left defenceless and susceptible to microbial invasion.

The normal acid mantle for skin and hair has a pH of between 4.0 and 5.9 (see also page 33). Once the pH rises above 6.5 bacterial invasion increases dramatically. Excess sunlight, poor diet, excessive sweating and strongly alkaline skin/hair products, soap or detergents can easily strip away the acid mantle. Citric and lactic acid are often incorporated into personal care products to help lower their pH and make them 'pH balanced'.

● ●

SKIN CARE TIP **AVOID HARSH SKIN PRODUCTS**

People with oily or acne-prone skin may mistakenly use overly aggressive cleansing techniques or highly alkaline products that strip the surface of oils needed to protect and waterproof the skin. This leaves the skin red, irritated and inflamed and vulnerable to damage. Apply a mineral-rich facial mask, or cleanse your skin with a micro-fibre facial cloth, to gently absorb excess surface oils without stripping away the protective acid mantle.

● ●

organic skin care products

More and more of us are committing to eating organic foods and using natural health remedies. But many people don't apply the same logic to the skin and still buy trendy high-street cosmetic brands without considering what goes into them.

Over the last 50 years, tens of thousands of new chemicals have been introduced. You are absorbing a vast array of these synthetic chemicals from food, toiletries and the environment. It is not only the danger of individual chemicals that is of concern but also their synergistic or 'cocktail' effect. At present we have no idea what the long-term effect of these chemical cocktails will be on us and our bodies. One Scandinavian trial showed that two preservatives are 1,000 times more toxic when occurring together than when used separately.

but is it organic?

It is not easy to be a green consumer. Almost every skin care product on the market today describes itself as 'natural', 'pure' or 'organic'. In fact, there can be thousands of different chemicals in natural toiletries, many of them synthetic.

There is currently no European Union (EU) legislation relating to the certification of cosmetics and personal care products made using organic ingredients – existing EU organic standards relate to foods and drinks only – however, several certification bodies set their own standards. To be sure that you are buying genuine organic skin care products, look out for the organic symbols from accredited certification bodies. As each organisation has drawn up its own standards, there may be individual differences between them, but the good news is that UK standards are recognised as the highest in the world.

● ●

DID YOU KNOW? **TOXIC OVERLOAD**

Man-made chemicals help manufacturers create cheap products with great skin-feel but with little skin care benefit, and just add to your toxic burden. The average woman uses 15 personal care products a day. Up to 60 per cent of the chemicals you put on your skin can end up in your bloodstream so you could be absorbing as much as 2kg of man-made chemicals every year!

● ●

organic certification

In the UK 'Organic Certification' means a product has been independently approved as meeting a specific standard. You are guaranteed that certified organic ingredients are used wherever they are available and that all ingredients are environmentally friendly (biodegradable) and free from genetically modified ingredients (GMOs).

There are three UK certification bodies (see page 219 for contact details and logos):

※ **Soil Association** was the first organisation to launch an organic standard for personal care products in May 2002.

※ **Non-food Certification Company** is a subsidiary of the Organic Food Federation and also launched an organic standard for personal care launched in 2002.

※ **UK Farmers & Growers** certifies organic personal care products under its food standards.

These groups have two levels of certification. Products containing over 95 per cent of agricultural ingredients from certified organic sources can include the word 'organic' in their title. Products made with between 70 per cent and 95 per cent agricultural ingredients from certified organic sources must indicate which ingredients are organic and say what percentage these comprise of the total.

There are other organic certifying bodies in Europe:

※ **Ecocert** is the largest certifying body in Europe and has two different product standards: 'natural' and 'organic'. The standards for 'natural' products are lower but, confusingly, the same symbol is used for both.

※ **BDIH** is the Federation of German Industries and Trading Firms in the fields of Cosmetics, Dietary Supplements and Nutritional Foods. The standards are for natural products (not organic) with the emphasis on the sourcing of ingredients from natural origins.

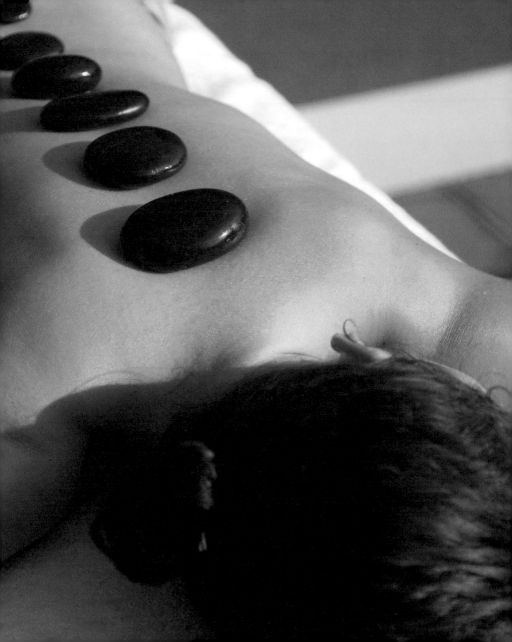

what's in your moisturiser?

There are a number of factors that limit the choice of ingredients that can be used in organic skin care products, which makes it difficult to create totally organic formulations. Currently, only salves, butters and balms can be 100 per cent organic. These products contain plant-based oils, waxes, essential oils and nothing else. As they don't contain water they don't need preservatives but consumers may find them heavy and greasy.

Water is the main ingredient of most skin care lotions and creams, accounting for as much as 75 per cent of the total. It may be listed as 'aqua' (Latin for water) or indicated by ingredients such as aloe vera juice, herbal infusions, seaweed extracts or floral waters.

Lighter skin care products such as creams and lotions are more complicated to formulate as water and oil must be held together by emulsifier. In addition, any product containing water needs a preservative to prevent it becoming contaminated with micro-organisms.

emollients

Emollients are the oily or fatty part of the emulsion. Emollients prevent dryness and protect the skin, providing lasting lubrication and softening. Natural emollients such as plant oils and butters are soluble in sebum, and easily absorbed and utilised by skin cells. They are readily biodegradable, available as organic ingredients and are of edible quality.

Most high-street skin care products use synthetic emollients such as mineral oils (paraffin wax and petrolatum) because they are cheap and stable. Mineral oils simply coat the skin, which stops the skin breathing and can cause irritation.

Other synthetic emolients include silicones (methicone and dimethicone). Like mineral oils they can inhibit the skin's ability to release toxins and may cause irritation. They are also non-biodegradable.

humectants

Skin creams are designed to keep skin moist and so must have humectant properties to retain skin moisture. Humectants draw and hold onto moisture from anything around them.

Collagen, elastin and keratin are widely used humectants as they are compatible with the skin and deposit a protective film. However, they are usually sourced from animals, and so most consumers prefer to avoid them.

Glycerine and lecithin are natural, plant-derived humectants. Glycerine, the most common, is derived from oils and fats made during soap-making. Natural phospholipids such as lecithin are excellent humectants as they increase skin hydration without forming a coating and so allow the skin to breathe.

Synthetic humectants such as propylene glycol can cause irritation and should be avoided.

detergents

Detergents are foaming emulsifiers found in shampoos, shower
gels and soaps. They're designed to emulsify oily grime, keeping it
in liquid suspension until it is washed away. Because all detergents
emulsify oils, they can remove sebum, leading to dry skin. They
can also interact with cell membranes, causing irritation.

Some detergents are more irritating than others. Harsh
detergents such as sodium lauryl sulphate (see page 189) strip
away natural protective oils, leaving the skin dry and inflamed.
Milder detergents such as coco betaine and decyl glucoside are
less irritating and are more suitable for sensitive skin.

colorants

Natural, nutrient-rich colours can be found in avocado, pumpkin
seed oil or chlorophyll (green), azulene from chamomile (blue) and
rose hip or calendula oils (golden orange). These colours are not as
vivid and vibrant as those from synthetic colours and may change
or fade with exposure to light and oxygen.

Avoid synthetic colours: they are used to make products look
more appealing to consumers but they can cause allergic skin
reactions. Some contain heavy metals and may be carcinogenic.

fragrance

As much as 95 per cent of the ingredients in the fragrances or
perfumes used in skin care products are synthetic. Fragrances are
a major cause of allergic reactions.

Blends of pure, natural essential oils provide a pleasant fragrance, but with added therapeutic properties. Scents made with natural ingredients may cause skin irritation, but you are less likely to suffer allergic reactions than with synthetic fragrances.

preservatives

Just like food, all natural skin care products eventually deteriorate and become unfit for use. Most cosmetics contain preservatives to prevent bacterial and fungal contamination during their intended shelf life. Preservatives are a leading cause of allergy and irritation. In particular, the following can cause allergic reactions or irritation, or may act as as donors of formaldehyde, a known carcinogen and neurotoxin: Methylchloroisothiazolinone, Methylisothiazolinone, 2-bromo-2-nitropropane-1,3-diol, diazolidinyl urea, DMDM hydantoin, imidazolidinyl urea, quaternium 15.

parabens

Parabens (including methyl, propyl, butyl and ethyl paraben) are commonly used as preservatives in personal care products. Although parabens are found in nature, they should be used with caution because they can disrupt hormone levels.

Research from the University of Reading published in 2004 found higher than normal levels of parabens in tissue from breast tumours. Research published in 1998 showed that butylparaben is the most powerful of these oestrogen-mimics, while propylparaben can reduce sperm production.

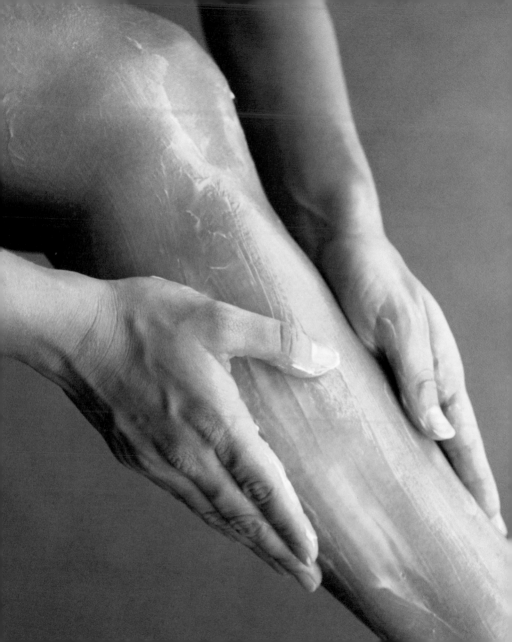

lanolin

Derived from sheep's wool, lanolin itself is perfectly safe and may be beneficial to the skin. But cosmetic-grade lanolin can be contaminated with carcinogens, such as the pesticide lindane, and organophosphates, which have been linked to central nervous system disorders.

talc

The cosmetic talc found in baby powders, face powders, body powders and some contraceptives is carcinogenic. Inhaling talc and using it in the genital area is associated with an increased risk of lung and ovarian cancer respectively. Talc should never be used on babies, both because of its carcinogenicity and due to the acute respiratory distress from inhalation that can result in death.

● ●

DID YOU KNOW? **SKIN DETOX**

When switching to organic skin care products, you might experience a 'skin detox'. Natural beauty therapists consider this a period of adjustment – your skin is in the process of cleansing itself of man-made chemicals. Be patient: it may take two to three weeks before you see a visible difference in your skin. This skin detox can be greatly assisted by undergoing an internal detox (see pages 42-3).

● ●

how safe is your deodorant?

Deodorant either masks the smell of stale sweat or inhibits the bacterial growth that causes it. Deodorants do not interfere with or inhibit the natural process of perspiring. Anti-perspirants, on the other hand, prevent sweating – a natural process vital to regulate temperature and eliminate toxins. So for the sake of your health avoid using anti-perspirants.

Concerns over the safety of deodorants and anti-perspirants are mainly due to the ingredients they may contain.

" Red meat is the number one cause of body odour. Shift to a healthy diet rich in vegetables, fresh fruit, seeds, nuts and omega fatty acids to clean up your body from the inside out. "

aluminium chloride/aluminium chlorohydrate

When applied to the skin, these chemicals enter the pores and form a thick gel that blocks the sweat glands. They have a tiny molecular size and readily penetrate the skin to enter the bloodstream, increasing levels of aluminium in the body. Higher levels of aluminium have been linked to several health problems affecting the central nervous system, including Alzheimer's disease.

alcohol (ethanol/ethyl alcohol)

As well as having a drying effect on the skin, ethanol often increases skin sensitivity and acts as a carrier, transporting other chemicals across the skin and into the bloodstream. The use of alcohol in cosmetics may therefore increase the absorption of other chemicals that come into contact with your skin, adding to the toxic burden in your body.

safe alternatives

Safe and effective alternatives include the mineral ammonium alum or alunite, and extracts from the castor oil plant, such as zinc ricinoleate, which have been used safely for centuries. Together, these two mineral salts prevent the growth of the bacteria responsible for body odour, and do not interfere with the vital process of perspiration.

● ●

SKIN CARE TIP **TRY A NATURAL PRE-DEODORANT**

If you suffer from strong body odour, mix equal parts of organic apple cider vinegar and water and pat onto your armpits. Wait until it has dried before applying your deodorant.

● ●

base oils for skin care

Natural ingredients should play an important part in your daily and weekly skin care programme. There are two main types: base oils can be used on their own as emollients to smooth, soften and moisturise the skin, while essential oils (see pages 82–5) can be mixed with base oils to provide special therapeutic properties.

The fatty acids that make up the structure of base oils give them powerful emollient (smoothing and softening) properties. Every base oil has a different combination of fatty acids, giving them individual properties suited to different uses. The following are the most popular and versatile base oils used in skin care:

avocado oil (*persea gratissima*)
This oil is rich in omega-6 linoleic acid, proteins, lecithin and vitamins A, B and D to nourish the skin. It can also be used as a hair grooming aid to give glossy and healthy hair. Its softening and rejuvenating properties help stop skin drying out.

coconut oil (*cocus nucifera*)
Coconut oil contains mainly saturated fatty acids and is therefore solid at room temperature. It protects the hair against sun damage, prevents and treats split ends and keeps it shiny and healthy. It is especially suitable for dry and sensitive skin.

cranberry oil (*vaccinium macrocarpon*)

This oil's unique natural balance of omega-3, 6 and 9 fatty acids and high level of natural antioxidants, especially tocotrienols (a form of vitamin E), aids the absorption and utilisation of essential fatty acids in the skin. Light and non-greasy, it easily penetrates and moisturises the skin. It is suitable for all skin types and may help relieve itchy, scaly, irritated skin conditions such as eczema and psoriasis.

evening primrose oil (*oenothera biennis*)

This oil is rich in beneficial plant sterols including beta-sitosterol, and unsaturated fatty acids gamma linoleic acid (GLA), essential for maintaining cell walls and reinforcing the immune system. It is suitable for all skin types, helping to nourish and revitalise skin tissues.

hemp seed oil (*cannabis sativa*)

Hemp seed oil is made up of 80 per cent essential fatty acids and contains the ideal ratio of omega-3 and 6, a combination that moisturises the skin without being greasy. It is added to hair products to treat hair and scalp conditions. It is suitable for all skin types, but its soothing and healing properties make it especially valuable for dry, eczema-prone and irritated skin. (Note: hemp oil is derived from a strain of *Cannabis sativa* that does not contain cannabinoids associated with the recreational drug.)

jojoba oil (*simmondsia chinensis*)

Jojoba oil is a liquid wax that closely resembles natural sebum. It also has anti-bacterial properties. It is a great base for essential oil blends and makes an excellent hair conditioner. It suits all skin types, but especially mature skin.

olive oil (*olea europaea*)

Olive oil has long been used for hair grooming and protection against sunburn and is often added to anti-wrinkle and eye creams, body lotions, hand creams, lip balm and creams. Rich in mono-unsaturates, it nourishes and protects the skin and prevents drying and so is ideal for dry and sensitive skins.

pomegranate oil (*punica granatum*)

Pomegranate oil contains over 80 per cent unsaturated fatty acids (including the unique punicic acid) and is rich in antioxidant polyphenols. This combination moisturises, nourishes and balances skin pH as well as neutralising free radicals. It helps repair and rejuvenate skin, smooth fine lines and wrinkles and improve elasticity. An excellent oil for eczema, psoriasis and mature, sunburned or ageing skin and acne.

rose hip oil (*rosa moschata*)

Rose hip oil's high concentration of natural vitamin E, linoleic (omega-6) and alpha-linolenic (omega-3) acids and other unsaturated fatty acids gives it outstanding medicinal properties. It is ideal for dry and mature skin and is clinically proven to heal cuts, treat scar tissue, nourish and relieve sensitive skin, promote cell regeneration and reduce the appearance of fine wrinkles.

" Base oils contain vitamins, minerals and essential fatty acids and can be highly effective in treating irritated, sensitve skin conditions, as well as helping to reduce wrinkles and scar tissue. "

sunflower oil (*helianthus annuus*)

Unrefined sunflower oil is very high in omega-6 fatty acids and a good source of vitamins and minerals, especially vitamin E. Sunflower oil is often used as a base for macerating (soaking) medicinal herbs so that the plant's active healing properties are transferred to the oil. This very light oil is suitable for all skin types. When used to macerate calendula (marigold), it has powerful healing and soothing properties for eczema, psoriasis and other irritated conditions.

essential oils for skin care

Essential oils contain the concentrated 'essence' of a plant – its active constituents, healing properties and energy as well as its scent. They are extracted from the flowers, leaves, fruit, peel, seeds, wood, bark or roots. Most are produced by steam distillation, some by pressing or solvent extraction. There are hundreds of essential oils, each with unique properties and characteristics.

Essential oils are highly concentrated – it takes 2,000 roses to produce one 10ml bottle of rose otto oil – so only tiny amounts are needed, usually 10–20 drops in 100ml of cream or lotion. They are highly volatile and evaporate easily and so are readily absorbed by the skin. Many personal care products contain essential oils that have been blended for their therapeutic properties, and not just their scent. The following are ten of the most popular and versatile essential oils used in skin care:

● ●

DID YOU KNOW? **ESSENTIAL OILS AND HEALTH**

Essential oils can enter the bloodstream to have therapeutic effects on internal organs such as the gut, lungs and kidneys.

● ●

bergamot (*citrus bergamia*)

Derived from the peel and pith of the bergamot orange, this sweet scented oil has calming and uplifting effects. It reduces oiliness and treats acne and spots.

Caution: unrefined bergamot oil contains bergapten, which forms a toxin in the presence of sunlight. In personal care products, it is important to use refined bergamot oil that is labelled 'bergapten-free'.

lavender (*lavandula angustifolia*)

A highly versatile oil with calming and soothing properties, lavender relaxes mind and body. A similar oil lavandin (*Lavandula hybrida super*) has similar properties but a sharper scent.

Lavender reduces inflammation and aids healing. It can be applied undiluted to small areas of skin; simply dab on spots and insect bites to speed healing.

mandarin (*citrus reticulata*)

A calming, soothing oil, mandarin is ideal for use on children and during pregnancy. It helps promote cell regeneration and prevent stretch marks in pregnancy. It is used to treat oily skin conditions, including acne, and can be applied directly to blackheads.

myrrh (*commiphora myrrha*)

Obtained by steam distillation of the resin in the myrrh bush, this is of the oldest scents known. It has refining and soothing properties, is ideal for mature complexions and helps to heal infected, cracked or chapped skin.

neroli (*citrus aurantium*)

Exotic neroli is distilled from the flowers of the bitter orange tree. Its sweet, floral aroma creates a feeling of euphoria and helps calm excited mental states. Neroil is great for all skin types and ages, but particularly mature skin, inflammation, irritation or redness. It tones the complexion and reduces thread veins.

roman chamomile (*anthemis nobilis*)

When freshly distilled, this oil is a delicate pale blue and has calming, soothing properties. It is used for reddened or inflamed conditions, such as eczema, dermatitis and psoriasis, spots and acne, and to heal wounds without scarring.

rose geranium (*pelargonium graveolens*)

Its heady aroma of sweet roses has a calming and revitalising effect on the senses. Suitable for use on all skin types, it balances sebum production and helps heal inflamed skin.

rosemary (*rosmarinus officinalis*)

This oil's stimulating and rejuvenating effects help alleviate stress-related disorders, such as nervous exhaustion, and ease headaches. It stimulates circulation in the scalp to treat greasy hair and scalp, dermatitis, psoriasis and dandruff.

sandalwood (*santalum austrocaledonicum*)

The heady, woody aroma of this oil is long lasting, exotic and sensuous, helping to calm and focus the senses. A great balancer of the skin, it is suitable for all skin types.

Caution: the traditional source of sandalwood (*Santalum album*) is becoming scarce due to over-harvesting in its native India. Oils derived from trees that are being sustainably grown in Australasia can be used with a clear conscience.

ylang ylang (*cananga odorata*)

Ylang ylang ('flower of flowers' in Malay) has a sensuous, sweet-floral scent. Long considered an aphrodisiac, it calms the mind, eases tensions and removes inhibitions. It is good for all skin types, but especially for oily, congested, inflamed or irritated skin.

face

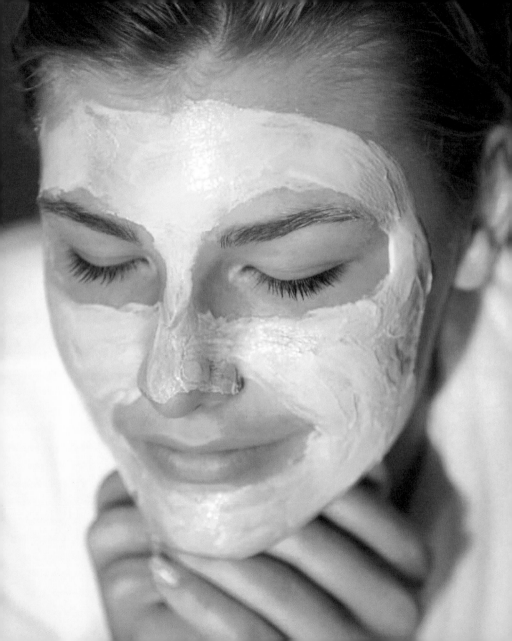

what your face reveals

Your face is a mirror of your mind, and of your general health. The different parts of your face reveal your state of health, and your facial expressions readily disclose your emotional state. Your skin also reveals your lifestyle. Extreme dryness could indicate a poor diet, low in essential fatty acids, while premature ageing could be caused by excessive sun exposure or smoking.

Your face also reveals the state of the internal organs. A red, bulbous, greasy nose, possibly with prominent veins, may indicate high blood pressure, heart and liver disorders or excess alcohol consumption. Yellow skin can indicate disorders of the liver, gallbladder, spleen and pancreas. Pale face and cheeks may indicate weak glands, congested and inactive liver, and/or anaemia. Cracks at the corners of the mouth can show vitamin B2 deficiency and digestive disorders.

" According to ancient healing systems such as ayurveda and traditional Chinese medicine, different parts of your face mirror the health of different organ systems. "

SKIN CARE TIP **FIND THE ROOT OF THE PROBLEM**

Skin care can only do so much to repair the damage caused by lifestyle and health problems. Always look for an underlying cause for skin problems by reviewing your diet (see pages 12-13 and 20-57) and factors such as excess sun exposure (see pages 115 and 212) and smoking, and seek your doctor's advice if any aspects of your health concern you.

caring for your complexion

If you want a naturally beautiful complexion, it is important to set aside some time each day to pamper and nourish your skin with natural organic skin care products, packed with plant-based nutrients and enzymes, and avoid chemical-laden branded creams and lotion that add to your body's toxic overload. Not sure of your skin type? Take the skin test on www.greenpeople.co.uk/skintest.

skin care basics

Your skin changes from day to day, depending on the season, weather, indoor climate, health and your physical and emotional wellbeing. It even alters between day and night (see page 93). To cater for these changes you may need to use different products for the different 'moods' of your skin. To get the best possible complexion, never stint on your skin care routine.

cleansing

Cleansing your face thoroughly – especially before bedtime – is essential to remove daily dirt, oil, grease and airborne pollution. Even foundation lotions and colour cosmetics are skin pollutants that can have a harmful effect if not removed regularly. Thorough cleansing stimulates the blood circulation to replenish the nutrients the skin needs and helps your skin absorb facial moisturisers better.

Cleansing must be deep enough to be effective, but very gentle to avoid damaging or drying your skin. Your skin acts as a barrier; over-cleansing not only strips off the dirt, grime and dead cells but also removes the oils that keep it healthy and balanced.

✳ Cleanse for at least a minute or two, twice a day.
✳ Choose the correct cleanser for your skin's mood – choices include semi-solid cleansing balms, thick cleansing creams, light lotions, milks, gels, soaps and cleansing wipes.

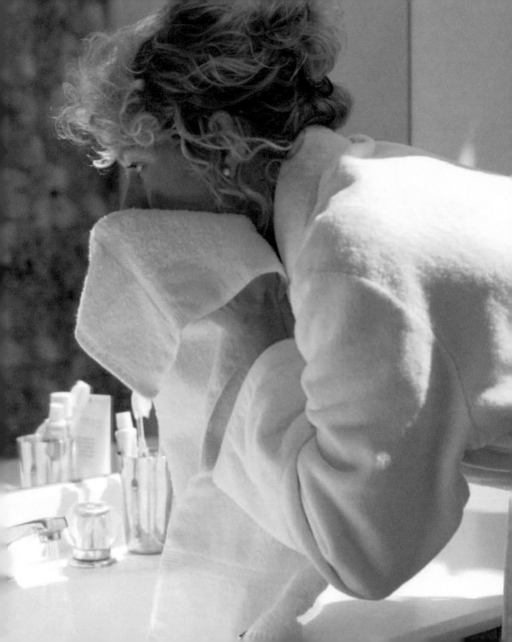

* Don't wash your face with very hot or ice cold water – both damage tiny blood vessels, or capillaries, in the skin.
* Don't use cleansers containing alcohol (ethanol/ethyl alcohol) – they strip the skin of essential oils.

● ●

DID YOU KNOW? **CLEANSING AND OILY SKIN**

Those with oily skin are prone to obsessive cleansing to get rid of the sheen. But this is counter-productive as cleansing more than twice a day actually increases oil production (see pages 100–2).

● ●

exfoliating

Many people skip this step in their skin care routine yet it brings an almost instant difference. By exfoliating your skin regularly you remove excess dead skin cells, and this immediately improves your skin's texture and appearance as it allows younger cells to come to the surface. Like cleansing, exfoliating improves circulation, helps skin absorb moisturisers and gives your complexion a healthy glow.

* Exfoliate once or twice a week.
* Choose a mineral based facial mask or a very gentle exfoliator to help remove the top layer of dead skin cells.
* Use a gentle scrub with tiny grains.
* Avoid cheap scrubs with large grains that will tear the skin.

toning

Some people swear by toners (facial mists), but many beauty experts do not. Toners remove the remaining traces of oil, makeup, dirt and cleanser, and hydrate the skin prior to applying moisturisers, creams and lotions. But for many skin types, using a good cleanser followed by splashing with cold water can do this just as well. A natural, plant-based toner strengthens your skin to give a better, smoother appearance, reduce visible fine wrinkles and restore its pH balance (see pages 33 and 64–5).

* Use a floral water-based facial mist – especially on a hot day, or to counteract the drying effect of central heating or when travelling or experiencing hot flushes.
* Avoid alcohol-based astringent toners – they're too harsh for your skin.

● ●

DID YOU KNOW? **YOUR SKIN BY DAY AND NIGHT**

During the day, your skin produces extra oil to protect itself from temperature changes, dirt and micro-organisms, as well as oxidation caused by UV light and pollutants. During the night your skin 'breathes' to rid itself of waste as well as repair any damage caused during the day.

● ●

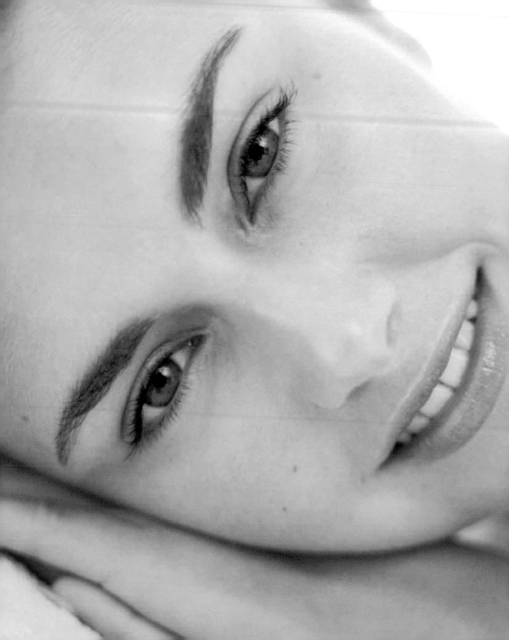

moisturising

With the possible exception of acne sufferers, everyone should moisturise – no matter what their skin type. Moisturising seals moisture into the skin and supports normal skin function. Your skin will tell you how much you should use. When your skin is tight, it's crying out for moisture. The perfect moisturiser will not feel greasy and should never irritate or burn.

Natural oil production also varies with your menstrual cycle, more oil being produced in the days before your period. Getting the balance right is important. Dry skin becomes thinner, loses elasticity, has poorer blood-circulation, less resistance to micro-organisms and inflammatory substances, and is more prone to eczema, psoriasis, allergies and the damaging effects of UV-rays.

* Always apply your moisturiser immediately after cleansing and toning, when the skin is still moist. The plant oils in the moisturiser can then trap the moisture in the skin. This is especially important for older skin as collagen and elastin fibres are less efficient at retaining moisture as we age.
* Don't over moisturise, as this causes clogged pores.
* Don't use a heavy moisturiser at night: it could prevent your skin ridding itself of waste. If your skin feels tight or dry, use a facial oil based on jojoba and/or rose hip followed by a light serum, or try a night treat containing natural fruit acids.

makeup safety tips

European legislation means that all cosmetic products with a shelf life of more than 30 months must indicate how long they can be used after opening. So we now know when to throw out old foundation, eye pencils, mascara and so on – but do we? And what about your foundation sponge and makeup brushes? Here are some tips…

makeup sponges and brushes

A moist environment is a perfect breeding ground for germs. A foundation sponge or brush mops up excess oils and impurities from spots, so bacteria can grow.

* Wash your foundation sponge after each use.
* Buy several makeup sponges, so you always have a dry, clean one when needed.
* Cleanse and condition your brushes once a week with a mild, natural soap or shampoo. Try natural organic soap with extracts of manuka and tea tree, which have powerful anti-microbial properties.
* Use a mild conditioner after washing the brushes, to ensure the softness of the brittle hairs, then rinse again in cold water. Remove excess water and dry flat on a towel.

mascara and eye pencils

Each time the mascara wand touches the eyelashes it picks up bacteria and transfers them to the tube. Preservatives in the product help prevent germs breeding, but may not cope with repeated bacterial contamination over a long period of time. Eye pencils trap bacteria, too, so take care not to scratch the eyeball.

* Replace your mascara every three months.
* Never share mascara with a friend.
* Always buy new mascara after recovering from an eye infection.
* Apply eye pencil outside the lash line.
* Keep pencils sharpened to shed the bacteria-laden wood casing.

" Always throw away your makeup if the colour changes or if it develops an odour. Preservatives degrade over time and may no longer be able to fight bacteria. "

lipgloss and lipstick

Lipgloss and lipstick harbour and pass on diseases, including viral infections such as Herpes simplex, which causes cold sores.

* Never leave the lid off your lipgloss/lipstick, as this encourages bacterial growth.
* Never share lipgloss or lipstick with a friend – especially if you have cold sores.

normal/combination skin

Normal skin is constantly renewing, healing and moisturising itself in a balanced way. This type of skin has an even tone and a smooth texture, free from greasy patches or flaky areas, and there are no visible pores or blemishes. Normal skin has an inner glow that stems from good blood circulation and excellent health. You may notice the occasional pimple just before your period, as increased hormonal activity over-stimulates the sebaceous glands.

If the skin on your forehead and around your nose (the 'T-zone') is oily while the rest of your face is normal or dry, you have combination skin. Your skin may be aggravated by changes in the weather, climate, diet, exercise and emotional wellbeing.

caring for normal skin

* Clean twice a day with a gentle, nourishing cleanser.
* After cleansing, tone with a mild alcohol-free toner such as a rosewater-based facial mist or a splash of cold water.
* Moisturise with a little light, organic facial cream. (Using moisturiser under makeup will help retain surface moisture.)
* At night time, if your skin feels tight, use a tiny amount of light organic facial cream or serum after cleansing and toning.
* Once a week, exfoliate your skin to stimulate the blood circulation, remove dead skin cells and smooth the surface of the skin. (See also page 92.)

caring for combination skin

❋ Use a gentle cleanser that does not leave skin feeling tight or dry.

❋ Avoid bar soaps or bar cleansers of any kind, regardless of the maker's claims. The ingredients are always more drying than those used in a gentle cleansing lotion.

❋ Apply an oil-absorbing facial mask as needed over oily areas.

❋ Opt for a water-based toner containing antioxidants and water-binding agents.

❋ Treat dry areas (including around the eyes) with a moisturiser containing antioxidants, water-binding agents and ingredients that mimic the structure and function of healthy skin. A serum-type product may be all your dry areas need to look and feel better. More extreme dryness will benefit from an antioxidant-rich serum paired with an emollient moisturiser.

● ●

SKIN CARE TIP **USE A T-ZONE MASK**

Mix 2 tablespoons of rosewater with 1 tablespoon of natural yoghurt and 1 tablespoon of manuka honey. If you wish you can add an essential oil from the chart on pages 130-1. Apply the mix to the T-zone, leave for 8-10 minutes and then rinse off.

● ●

oily skin

This type of skin has hyperactive sebaceous glands, working overtime to produce excess oils and sebum, and cellular renewal is speeded up too. This results in shiny skin, visible pores, pimples, blemishes, acne and inflammation. Oily skin can be due to poor diet, fluctuating hormone levels, hormonal contraceptives and choice of cosmetics. Humidity and hot weather can make the skin even greasier.

The flow of sebum or oil often increases during adolescence, pregnancy and after the menopause, again because of hormonal changes. The problem can occur at any age but tends to decrease with age. One advantage of oily skin is that it ages at a slower rate than other skin types.

● ●

SKIN CARE TIP **MIST TO KEEP MAKEUP IN PLACE**

To prevent the problem of your makeup becoming patchy, either on the forehead, chin or nose due to excessive oiliness in these areas, apply a rosewater facial mist on the excessively oily parts of your face, dry thoroughly and then apply your makeup.

● ●

caring for oily skin

❋ Use plenty of warm (not hot) water and a gentle, yet effective cleanser to stop the pores clogging. A foam-based anti-bacterial cleanser that is organic and rich in active plant nutrients reduces the risk of cleanser-induced skin irritation.

❋ Avoid astringent lotions and irritating alcohol-based toners that strip the skin of natural oils. Your oil glands will just work harder to compensate for the oils lost.

❋ Wash your face two or three times a day (morning and evening are essential), but no more or you will over-stimulate your skin to produce more oil.

❋ Always rinse your face thoroughly.

❋ Use a facial micro-fibre cloth or a muslin cloth, which works as a gentle exfoliator to dislodge dead skin cells and cleanse the pores. Remember to wash the cloth thoroughly every day.

❋ You can follow this with an alcohol-free facial mist to hydrate the skin.

❋ If your skin feels tight, apply a light moisturiser.

❋ Apply a deep-cleansing mineral mask twice a week.

❋ Never apply makeup unless your skin is thoroughly cleansed, and remove all traces of makeup before you go to bed.

diet for oily skin

❋ Eat plenty of leafy green vegetables and fresh fruits.

❋ A deficiency of vitamin B2 can cause oily skin. Good sources
  include brewer's yeast, whole grains, beans and nuts.

❋ Buckwheat, black beans and whole rice are rich in iron, which
  can rejuvenate the skin.

❋ Add plenty of omega-3 fatty acids to your diet (see pages 50–3).

❋ Drink lots of filtered water to both keep your skin hydrated
  and flush out toxins.

❋ Avoid saturated and hydrogenated fats, fried and highly seasoned
  foods, soft drinks, alcohol, sugar, chocolate and junk food.

● ●

SKIN CARE TIP **FILTER WATER**

If you suffer from acne, oily skin, acne rosacea or dry skin, it is a good idea
to buy a water filtering system that removes contaminants such as calcium,
chlorine, heavy metals and agricultural and industrial pollutants. These
systems also soften tap water, reducing the risk of sensitising the skin, and
are cost effective – detergents and foaming agents work more effectively in
soft water, so you' ll be able to use less of them, saving yourself money!
(For stockist see page 218.)

● ●

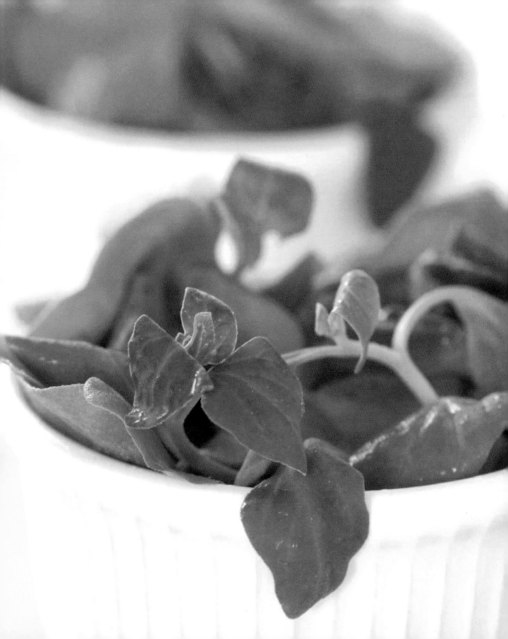

dry skin

A slowing down of sebum production results in dry, flaky and easily chapped skin. This problem is exacerbated by environmental factors such as strong sunshine, wind, cold, extremes of temperature (two-thirds of women in the northern hemisphere suffer from dry skin in the winter months), air conditioning, central heating, atmospheric pollutants and strong exfoliators, which strip the skin of moisture. Harsh cosmetics, alcohol-based personal care products and excessive bathing with strong detergents such as sodium lauryl sulphate (see page 189) all add to the problem.

Dry skin can also be a sign of dietary deficiencies, especially of essential fatty acids and vitamins A and B complex. Alcohol and caffeine are both diuretics and can dehydrate the skin. Dry skin can also be a sign of an under-active thyroid. Certain medications, such as diuretics and antihistamines contribute to dry skin.

caring for dry skin

* Avoid going from very hot to very cold environments.
* Keep rooms moist, especially in winter, by placing bowls of water by the radiators, or use a humidifier.
* Avoid excess exposure to strong sunshine, and apply a good sunscreen to exposed areas of your skin.

* Get plenty of sleep, as cellular repair is at its greatest when you are at rest.
* Regular exercise will nourish and cleanse your skin from within.
* Choose a gentle alcohol-free cleanser, such as an organic cleansing balm rich in nourishing oils.
* Avoid harsh exfoliators, strong detergents and very hot water.
* A soft facial cloth made from ultra-fine micro-fibres is better for the skin than a rough-textured washcloth, which can cause irritation to dry skin.
* Dry skin needs regular stimulation with massage and a balancing facial oil rich in ingredients such as rose hip and pomegranate.
* A quality natural moisturiser increases the water content of the skin and gives it a soft, moist look.
* Use a facial mist or pure mineral water to freshen your face during the day.
* Always apply moisturiser to face and neck with light, tapping, upwards motions while the skin is still slightly damp. This helps lock in moisture and stimulates the circulation.
* Before bed, use a very rich cleansing balm. Remove residue with a spray of facial mist. Follow with a tiny amount of facial oil and a facial serum. Once a week, use a facial mask to clarify the skin and remove dull, dry surface skin cells.

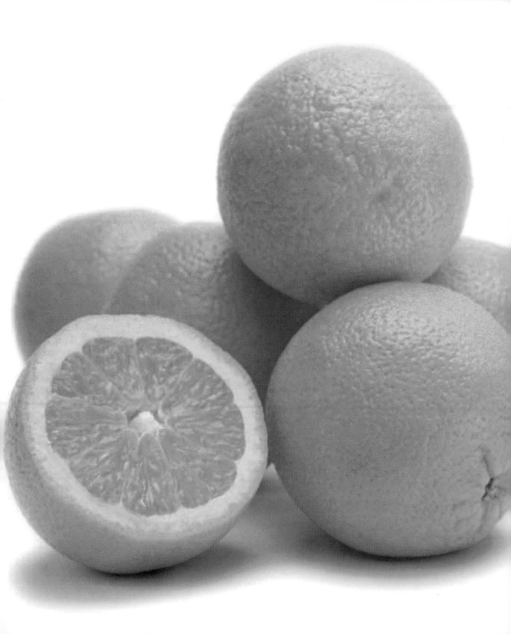

diet for dry skin

* Drink lots of filtered water and non-diuretic herbal teas.
* Limit alcohol and caffeine, which have a diuretic effect and can aggravate dry skin.
* Supplement your diet with vitamins, minerals and essential fatty acids from evening primrose oil.
* Snack on sunflower and pumpkin seeds and nuts.
* Include plenty of oily fish in your diet. Also try one of the many omega-3 and omega-6 essential oil blends, or buy unrefined, cold-pressed vegetable oil such as flax seed oil. These oils can be used daily on salads and baked potatoes, or mixed into cold dishes.
* Eat plenty of yellow and orange vegetables and fruits, rich in antioxidant vitamins C and beta-carotene, green leafy vegetables and wheat germ, sources of vitamin B5.
* Increase your intake of vitamin E (found in avocados, wholegrains, nuts and seeds), which is an antioxidant that protects the skin from ageing and maintains elasticity.
* Ensure your diet includes zinc, which is involved in hundreds of enzyme reactions essential for skin health. Natural sources include oysters and sesame and pumpkin seeds.
* Garlic, onions, eggs and asparagus are high in sulphur, which helps to keep the skin smooth and youthful.
* Avoid fried foods, animal fat and hydrogenated vegetable oils, which increase production of destructive free radicals.
* Avoid soft drinks, sugar, chocolate, crisps, or other junk foods.

sensitive skin

Sensitive skin is usually thin or fine-textured with blood vessels lying close to the surface. As a result, it is easily affected by chemical and atmospheric irritation leading to blotchiness, redness, dehydration and irritation. Sensitive skin is prone to dermatitis, acne, eczema, nettle rash, blackheads, rosacea or non-specific inflammation (erythema), dryness, stinging, itching or blistering.

Sensitive skin reacts to both heat and cold and so burns easily in the sun and wind. It is easily stimulated by stress, alcohol, spicy food and harsh climate, which all cause dilation of the fine blood vessels close to the skin surface as well as chronic dehydration and often irregular oil production. Cosmetics and skin treatments containing alcohol, perfume, detergents or other harsh ingredients can all cause irritation, leaving the skin red and blotchy.

SKIN CARE TIP **TEST FOR SENSITIVITY**

Before applying a new makeup or facial care product to your face, test it first by applying a little to the inside of your forearm. If no reaction is observed after an hour, apply it a second time to the same area and leave on for 12 hours. If there is no inflammation or irritation after this time it should be safe to use on sensitive skin.

" If you suffer from sensitive skin avoid wearing fake jewellery and synthetic fabrics. If you must wear perfume, spray it onto your clothes rather than applying it directly onto your skin. "

caring for sensitive skin

* Avoid saunas, steam or rubbing affected areas, which can exacerbate the problem.
* Install a water filter system (see page 102), as chlorine is a very common cause of skin problems.
* Room air filtration units can also be very helpful to clear the air of airborne allergens.
* Avoid harsh skin care products, including exfoliating scrubs and detergents such as sodium lauryl sulphate (see page 189). These can abrade the skin, making it more permeable to other irritants.
* Avoid products containing potential allergens such as synthetic fragrance. For those with extreme sensitivities, even natural essential oils can trigger a reaction. Natural unscented products are made specially for super-sensitive skin.
* Cleanse morning and evening with a gentle natural cleansing lotion, rinse thoroughly and pat the skin dry with a very soft towel. Follow with a light facial mist.
* In the morning apply a light moisturiser. In sunshine, use a moisturiser with built-in sun protection – SPF 15 is ideal.

hypoallergenic products

'Hypoallergenic' products are often recommended for sensitive skin, yet there is no legal definition of this term. Hypoallergenic usually means products do not contain synthetic fragrances, a leading cause of allergic sensitisation and contact dermatitis, resulting in reddened skin, stinging eyes and dryness. Products claiming to be hypoallergenic may contain formaldehyde-based preservatives, such as imidazolidinyl urea, diazolidinyl urea, quaternium-15, and DMDM hydantoin. These, too, can cause skin reactions. People with sensitive skin may want to avoid these ingredients.

diet for sensitive skin

* In some cases foods or food additives may cause skin irritation. If you suspect this is the case, seek an allergy test or visit a kinesiologist to identify the problem ingredient.
* Drink at least eight glasses of pure, filtered water daily to help your body detoxify.
* Increase your consumption of omega-3 fatty acids, found in oily fish and flax seed oil (see pages 50–3).
* Supplement your diet with evening primrose oil (rich in GLA) and vitamin C.
* Avoid too much spicy food and alcohol.
* Cut out junk food and avoid additives such as food colourings, as they can trigger inflammation.

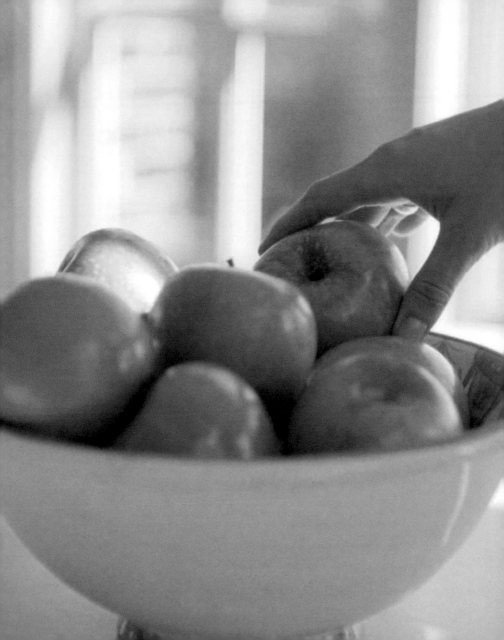

holding back the clock

The rate at which your skin changes with age depends on several factors, including your genes and your state of health. Natural, or intrinsic, ageing – the effects of gravity, hormonal changes and time itself – cannot be avoided. As we get older, the skin starts to wrinkle and sags at the neckline, causing deep smile lines and drooping eyebrows. Less sebum is produced, therefore the skin becomes drier. Moisture will evaporate more quickly from the skin cells causing dehydration.

But it's not just age that gives us lines; exposure to the sun, poor diet and nutrition, loss of muscle tone, smoking, increased stress and environmental changes all affect the condition of your skin. You can try to prevent your skin ageing prematurely by following a good skin care regime, eating healthily and protecting your skin from extrinsic factors such as the sun and cigarette smoke (yours and other people's). Even your sleeping position has an effect on how your skin ages.

intrinsic ageing

The signs of intrinsic ageing cannot be avoided and they tend to follow a set pattern:

❋ **0 to 15 years:** the skin texture is smooth, pores are small. The skin works very efficiently and easily retains water. There is no visible damage due to sun exposure. Hormonal changes during teenage years can lead to an increase in sebum secretion and the development of spots and acne.

* **15–25 years:** Spots and acne can be a real problem now. Tiny fine lines begin to appear and pore size is increasing. Sebaceous gland activity is high and cell turnover is still rapid. The skin's ability to retain water starts to decline.

* **25–45 years:** Fine lines are here to stay and the first wrinkles are appearing due to UV damage (see pages 115 and 212–13). Early signs of sagging appear near the eyes, and the skin is losing elasticity. The rate of loss of the old skin cells slows down, and the epidermis gradually becomes less translucent and does not retain water so well.

* **45–55 years:** More wrinkles now appear and, in most cases, skin texture becomes coarser. Pores and age spots enlarge and become more defined. Sagging near eyes and cheeks is now more apparent. There is a decrease in skin repair and immune system function and the epidermis becomes thinner. The skin tends to be dry.

* **55 years onwards:** Wrinkles and fine lines increase. The uneven colour, pigmentation and sagging increases. Dermal repair is reduced and production of collagen and sebum declines. Damage from sun exposure has been accumulating over many decades. Older skin looks drier, less radiant and less plumped out. This problem can affect all older people, but those who protect their skin from the sun tend to preserve the tone and structure of their complexion for longer.

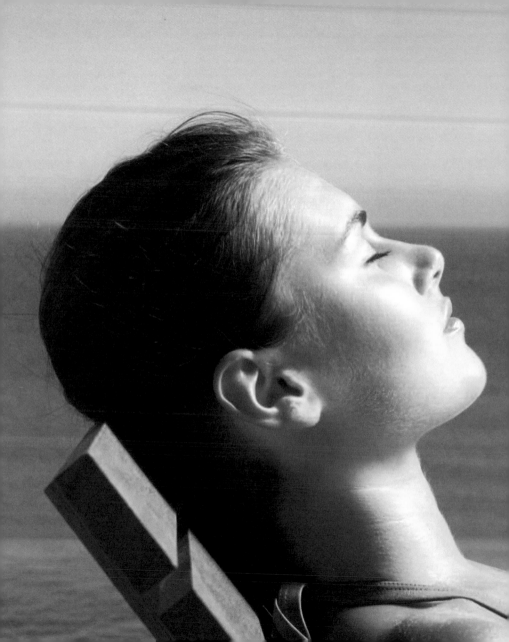

sun exposure

Some sun exposure is necessary for vitamin D production, and to prevent the 'winter blues' or Seasonal Affective Disorder (SAD). But most signs of premature skin ageing are due to excess sun over many years (known as photoageing). To protect your skin

❋ Avoid self-tanning with sun beds and sun lamps, including indoor tanning devices.

❋ Stay out of the sun between 11am and 3pm when the sun's rays are at their strongest.

❋ Wear a wide-brimmed hat and long sleeves when outdoors.

❋ All year round, apply broad spectrum sunscreen (UVA and UVB protection) with a sun protection factor (SPF) of 15.

" The amount of photoageing you develop depends on both your skin colour and your history of sun exposure. "

smoking

Cigarette smoking causes biochemical changes in our bodies that accelerate ageing. Research shows that a person who smokes 10 or more cigarettes a day for a minimum of 10 years is statistically more likely than a non-smoker to develop deeply wrinkled, leathery skin with a yellowish hue. However, these signs can be greatly diminished, and in some cases reversed, by stopping smoking. Even people who have smoked for many years show less facial wrinkling and improved skin tone when they quit.

sleeping positions

Resting your face on the pillow in the same way every night for years can lead to sleep lines. Over time, these lines become etched onto the skin and do not disappear when you get out of bed. Women who sleep on their sides are likely to see these lines appear on their chin and cheeks. People who sleep on their backs do not develop these wrinkles since their skin does not lie crumpled against the pillow.

caring for mature skin

* Limit your exposure to strong sunshine and use a cream with at least an SPF 8 or SPF 15, depending on skin type.
* Never use water that is too hot as it can dehydrate the skin and cause broken thread veins.
* Avoid irritating ingredients based on mineral oils, which can draw natural oils out of the skin, and products with a high alcohol content, which will make your skin feel even dryer.
* Cleanse your skin morning and evening.
* If your skin isn't too sensitive use a gentle exfoliator once a week to get rid of old, flaky skin cells. Never over-exfoliate mature skin as this can thin your skin even more.
* Use a moisturiser rich in active plant nutrients. Always apply your moisturiser to both face and neck with light tapping, upwards motions while your skin is still slightly damp, or have a stimulating facial massage. This helps to lock in moisture and also stimulates the blood circulation in the skin.

❋ Apply a non-drying moisturising face mask once a week –
ideally after a bath – to give your skin a well-deserved boost.
Leave the mask on for at least 20 minutes and then wipe it off
with a warm cloth.

● ●

SKIN CARE TIP **USE A REJUVENATING FACIAL OIL**

Try this rejuvenating facial oil – it is great for mature skin. Add 10–15 drops
of a suitable essential oil (see page 131), such as geranium or rose oil, to
30ml of base oil (such as apricot or rose hip). For example, try neroli for
dehydrated, sensitive skin and broken capillaries, patchouli to soothe dry
and inflamed skin and frankincense if you have wrinkles.

After hydrating the face with toner or a splash of cold water, apply the
oil sparingly over the whole face and neck with light tapping motions. Then
gently stroke the oil over the skin, starting at the base of the neck and
working upwards and outwards to the forehead and temples. Allow the oil
time to soak in, then blot off any excess with a clean tissue.

● ●

diet for mature skin

Drink lots of water and eat plenty of fresh, organic fruits and
vegetables, oily fish and/or flax seed oil, and eat brown rice at least
twice a week. These are easily digested and help eliminate the
toxins that contribute to premature ageing.

anti-ageing facial workout

As we age our facial muscles weaken and skin begins to sag. Just as gym workouts promote the body's youthful strength and suppleness, facial exercises strengthen facial muscles to improve circulation and revitalise tired skin, for example giving you a smoother, firmer neck.

Daily movements such as eating, talking and laughing aren't enough to promote facial fitness. The chin, neck, throat, lips and eyes, in particular, are difficult areas to treat, but regular facial exercises, to isolate and exercise the muscles of the face, chin and neck, can make you look years younger. Here is a quick and effective daily routine to try. Before you begin, wash your face and hands.

neck and throat

* Sit upright, tilt your head back and look up at the ceiling. With lips closed, make a chewing movement. You'll feel the muscles working in the neck and throat and will be truly amazed at the results. Repeat 20 times.

* Sit upright, tilt your head back and look up at the ceiling. Close and relax your lips, then pucker them in a kiss. Now stretch the kiss, as if trying to kiss the ceiling. Keep your lips puckered for a count of 10, and then relax, bring your head back to its normal position. Repeat five times.

cheeks

* Have a relaxed smile with your lips closed and then suck in your cheeks towards and on to your teeth. Hold this for a count of 10 and then relax. Repeat 10 times.
* Look in a mirror while doing the following exercise. Smile as broadly as possible while keeping your lips closed and mouth corners turned up. Try to make your mouth corners touch your ears. Next, wrinkle your nose and see your cheek muscles move upwards. Feel these muscles really work. Stay like this for a count of five and then relax. Repeat 10 times.

● ●

DID YOU KNOW? **EXERCISE SPOTS**

Minor spots or blemishes may appear after starting facial exercises because your skin is stimulated to produce extra oils and lubricants. These will disappear once your skin begins to function efficiently.

● ●

eyes

❋ To gently tone the muscles of the eyes, place two fingers on each side of your head, at the temples, and press while opening and closing your eyes rapidly. Repeat five times.

❋ Sit upright. While keeping your eyes closed and relaxed the whole time, look down and then look up as far as possible. Repeat this 10 times.

❋ Eye tapping can reduce crow's feet and puffiness. Tap gently with the pads of your fingers from the inside corner, near the nose, to the outer edge and back again, following the curve under the eye. Repeat 10 times.

forehead

❋ Frown as much as possible and try to bring your eyebrows over your eyes while also pulling them towards one another. Then lift your eyebrows as high as possible while opening your eyes as wide as possible. Repeat 5 times.

lips

❋ Sit upright facing forwards and keep your lips closed and teeth together. Smile as broadly as possible, without opening your lips. Keep like this for a count of five and then relax. Now pucker your lips into a pointed kiss. Keep like this for a count of five and then relax. Repeat 10 times.

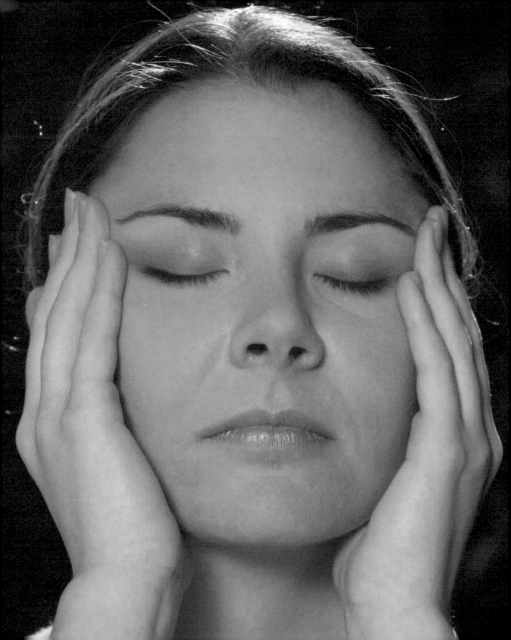

complexion problems

Many of us take a healthy complexion for granted, but some people are not so lucky and suffering from a facial skin condition can be very depressing. Caring for your skin, and indeed your whole body, is best achieved from the inside out – with some basic changes to your lifestyle, you should be able to improve your complexion dramatically.

ACNE

Acne is mainly due to over-active sebaceous glands. Excessive sebum, together with dead skin cells, can block hair follicles and pores. Sebum accumulates and feeds bacteria, leading to spots, pimples, white heads and blackheads. Acne mainly occurs on the forehead, cheeks and chin, but can appear on the neck, back and chest. It is most common during the teenage years, when hormone levels are fluctuating, but can break out at all stages of life.

skin care for acne

* Avoid harsh detergents or alcohol-based cleansers, synthetic fragrances and abrasive, grainy or chemical exfoliators.
* Use makeup sparingly to stop pores becoming clogged. Foundation sponges, blusher brushes and makeup brushes are a haven for bacteria and so need regular cleaning to avoid re-infection (see page 96).

✳ Change your face and hand towels daily and keep your hands clean.

✳ Choose a swept-back hair style and avoid having a fringe.

✳ Don't use hair-styling products as they can block follicles and irritate the skin.

✳ Cleanse your face twice daily using a gentle, natural cleanser rich in natural antibacterial agents such as tea tree and manuka (see page 90). Choose natural products containing soothing ingredients such as chamomile, marshmallow and calendula.

✳ Splash your face with cold water (use filtered water if your face is very sensitive) to stimulate the flow of blood to the skin surface, which improves the transport of healing nutrients and helps remove waste products.

✳ Use seaweed- and clay-based facial masks twice a week to help unblock pores and heal the skin.

✳ Try a facial sauna or steam bath with essential oils such as chamomile and sage, or use green tea and chamomile tea bags.

✳ Dab each acne spot with a cotton bud dipped in a blend of equal parts of lavender, chamomile, tea tree and myrrh. This reduces redness, swelling and pimples.

✳ Use an antibacterial spot-cover lotion containing zinc oxide.

✳ Add a few drops of milk to some ground nutmeg to form a paste, apply to the spots and leave on for 1–2 hours before rinsing away.

✳ Dab a little natural toothpaste on the pimples just before you go to bed. Leave on overnight and wash off in the morning.

* Alternatively, make a paste of honey and cinnamon powder, apply before you go to bed and wash off with warm water in the morning.
* Rub fresh garlic on and around the pimples and leave on for as long as possible.

● ●

DID YOU KNOW? **POPPING PIMPLES**

It is tempting to squeeze pimples to remove them but this can push bacteria deep into the skin, causing more severe inflammation and swelling. In addition, scabs may form, leading to scar tissue. You also risk damaging the pores so that they can't function.

● ●

diet for acne-sufferers

* Avoid deep-fried and fatty foods, processed foods, sugar, wheat-based bread and cereals, yeast, alcohol, cow's milk and cheese, artificial food preservatives and sweeteners, chocolate, coffee, cola and other carbonated drinks, oranges and orange juice, red meat, salty snacks, peanuts and spicy foods.
* Start the day with a large glass of lukewarm water and freshly squeezed lemon juice.
* Increase your intake of fresh, organic fruit and vegetables (avoid oranges).

- ❉ Eat plenty of fresh oily fish or supplement your diet with omega-3 and omega-6 oils (see pages 51–3).
- ❉ Snack on seeds and nuts – especially pumpkin, sunflower and almonds (avoid peanuts).
- ❉ Eat pulses, wholegrains such as rice, oats and rye and plain bio-yoghurt.
- ❉ Include plenty of cabbage, broccoli, Brussels sprouts, garlic, onions and ginger in your meals.
- ❉ Ensure your diet supplies plenty of the minerals zinc, magnesium, selenium and chromium and vitamin A to help speed healing and reduce soreness.
- ❉ Drink green tea after a meal to aid digestion and help detoxify your system, but don't add sugar as this neutralises the beneficial effects.
- ❉ Herbal remedies such as milk thistle can also be useful in promoting proper liver function to reduce overall toxin levels in the body.

" If you suffer from acne, try using a cleansing diet, such as the three-day detox programme (see pages 42–3), to get rid of the impurities in your system. "

ROSACEA

Rosacea is a chronic condition that can occur in the middle-aged. It is often referred to as 'adult acne'. The face becomes flushed due to dilation of small blood vessels close to the surface. It is often accompanied with severe dryness and irritation around the chin, cheeks, nose and forehead. Rosacea sufferers react badly to changes in temperature, as well as to alcohol, spicy meals, coffee, oranges and skin care products containing fragrances, alcohol and fruit acids.

skin care for rosacea

* Wear a natural sunscreen with an SPF 15 year round and keep your face cool, if possible, by staying in an air-conditioned environment on hot, humid days. Otherwise sip cold drinks or suck ice cubes or spray the face with cool water or rosewater-based toner.
* In cold weather cover your cheeks and nose with a scarf.
* Begin each day with a thorough and gentle facial cleansing. Use a gentle cleanser that is not grainy or abrasive and spread it with your fingertips. Rinse the face with lukewarm water to remove dirt and any remaining cleanser and use a thick cotton towel to gently blot the face dry.
* Use a gentle, natural moisturiser during cold weather to protect against the drying effects of cold and wind.
* Avoid hot water, hot tubs and saunas. These can bring on flushing and aggravate your condition.

⁕ Avoid rough washcloths, brushes or sponges. Select fragrance-free products or use products scented with organic essential oils, if your skin agrees.

● ●

SKIN CARE TIP **PRACTICE VISUALISATION**

Stress can trigger rosacea, so use deep-breathing exercises (see pages 16–17) and try the following visualisation technique. Sit in a quiet place, close your eyes and visualise a beautiful holiday spot or a favourite pastime. Hold the image for several minutes until the restful feeling it generates is really taking effect.

● ●

diet for rosacea

⁕ Avoid steaming hot soup, coffee, alcohol, hot spices such as pepper and spicy foods such as nachos.

⁕ Other foods that often trigger flare-ups include cheese, sour cream, yoghurt, citrus fruits, liver, chocolate, vanilla, soy sauce, yeast extract, vinegar, aubergines, avocados, spinach, broad-leafed beans and pods, and foods high in histamine or niacin.

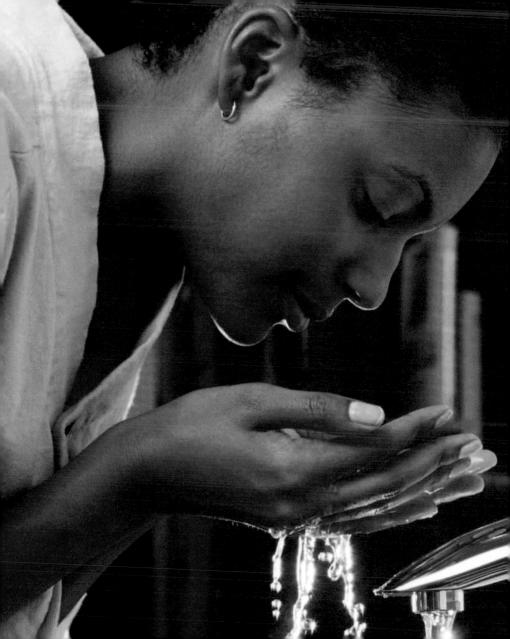

LARGE SKIN PORES

Skin pores are tiny openings through which sweat from the sweat glands and sebum (oil) from the sebaceous glands are secreted. Pores increase in size by up to 20 per cent in hot weather as they work overtime to release excess sweat and sebum.

If pores are not cleaned regularly, grease and dead skin can accumulate and they can become clogged, causing blemishes. Pores are not very elastic so once they are stretched, they tend not to shrink back to their younger, smaller state.

Skin pore size is also genetically determined. You can keep pores from getting bigger and make them appear smaller, but there is no cream, ointment or skin care regime that can actually shrink pores, although many products claim to. If you already have large pores, look at the positive side: your skin produces more oil so it is less likely to develop wrinkles than a dry, fine-textured complexion.

skin care for large pores

* Start by cleansing your face at least twice a day with a gentle cleanser, preferably in combination with an ultra-fine exfoliating micro-fibre cloth to gently draw dirt and grime away from your skin without stripping natural oils from your skin.
* Follow with a light moisturiser, facial gel or serum and avoid pore-clogging foundations.
* A weekly deep-cleansing treatment with a mineral-based mask helps maintain clear skin and stops pores from getting larger.

oils for your skin type

A few drops of essential oils in your homemade face mask or combined with a blend of base oils suitable for your skin type will provide a spa-like treat. As a golden rule never use more than 16-20 drops of essential oil mix per 100ml base oil. Figuring out which essential oils work best can be confusing. Below is a list of base and essential oils suitable for each main skin type. Oils such as olive, sunflower and palm are suitable for most skin types providing they are used in the right ratio in the formulation.

BASE OILS	ESSENTIAL OILS
normal skin (see page 98)	
Joboba, sesame, pomegranate	Rose geranium, Roman chamomile, fennel, lavender, patchouli, rose, sandalwood
combination skin (see pages 98–9)	
Joboba, hemp, pomegranate	Rosewood, ylang-ylang, rose geranium
oily skin (see pages 100–2)	
Melon seed, hemp, sunflower, evening primrose	Cedarwood, bergamot, rose geranium, clary sage, lemon, cypress, frankincense, juniper vetivert, grapefruit, lavender

dry skin (see pages 104–7)

Cocoa butter, rose hip oil, jojoba, coconut, sesame, hemp, pomegranate

Rose geranium, hyssop, patchouli, rose, roman chamomile, sandalwood, ylang-ylang

sensitive skin (see pages 108–10)

Rose hip, jojoba, calendula, olive, melon seed

Chamomile, rose, neroli, lavender, sandalwood

mature skin (see pages 116–17)

Grape seed, apricot, rose hip, jojoba, pomegranate, sesame

Frankincense, rose geranium, myrrh, rose, neroli, palmarosa

acne (see pages 122–5)

Pomegranate, hemp, melon seed, evening primrose

Tea tree, manuka, lavender, thyme, rose geranium, myrrh, grapefruit, bergamot, vetiver, juniper, lemongrass, German and Roman chamomile, cedarwood, palmarosa

rosacea (see pages 126–7)

Evening primrose, rose hip

German chamomile, rosewood, rose geranium

eczema (see pages 160–5)

Pomegranate, hemp, evening primrose, avocado

German and Roman chamomile, lavender, helichrysum, rose geranium, sandalwood

psoriasis (see pages 166–9)

Hemp, pomegranate, avocado

German or Roman chamomile, lavender, rose geranium, sandalwood

homemade skin treats

Many natural ingredients have special properties that help heal, soothe and rejuvenate the complexion. They can be made into effective facial recipes with little time and effort.

jojoba cleanser and eye makeup remover

Jojoba is non-greasy and rich in antioxidant vitamin E (tocopherols) giving it natural moisturising and healing properties. It is also resistant to oxidation and so very stable. Add 50ml jojoba oil to 6 drops of an essential oil or blend that suits your skin type (see pages 130–1). Store in an airtight bottle and use within four weeks. (For treating eczema, psoriasis and acne-prone skin use hemp seed oil.)

vinegar toner

Vinegar has a tonic action that promotes circulation in the tiny capillaries that nourish the skin. It is also antiseptic, dissolves excess fatty deposits on the skin surface, reduces scaly or peeling conditions, and regulates the skin's pH (see pages 33 and 65). Apple cider vinegar is rich in enzymes and organic acids and full of vitamins and minerals. It is particularly effective when used with lavender, rose or rosemary essential oils. Stir 1–2 tablespoons of apple cider vinegar into 250ml of water and add up to 5 drops of an essential oil or blend that suits your skin type. Apply to your face after cleansing. Keep refrigerated and use within four weeks.

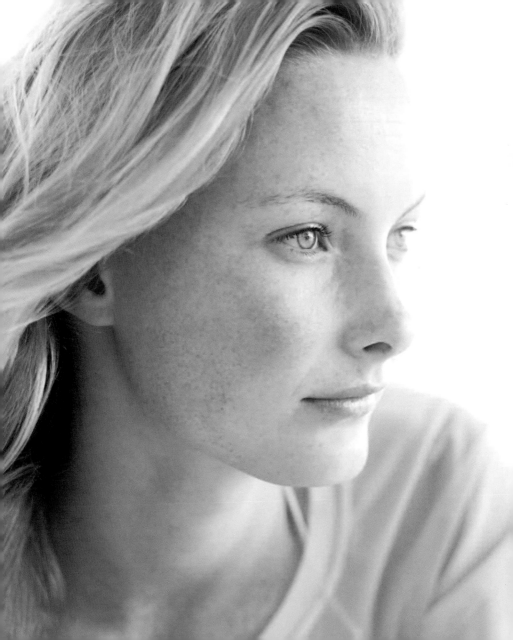

avocado mask with manuka honey

Avocado is rich in vitamins A, D and E, beta-carotene, potassium (the 'youth mineral'), proteins, lecithin and essential fatty acids. It also contains plant steroids called sterolins, which help soften and moisturise the skin, reduce age spots and heal sun damage and scars. Avocado is wonderfully emollient and assists in the regeneration and rejuvenation of the skin. It is ideal for mature, dehydrated and sun- or climate-damaged skin. It also helps relieve the dryness and itching of psoriasis and eczema.

All honey naturally attracts moisture and penetrates deeply, moisturising and repairing the cracking or damage caused by dryness. Manuka honey is highly antibacterial and rich in vitamins, minerals, proteins, enzymes and amino acids essential for healthy skin. Active manuka honey is unique to New Zealand and contains non-peroxide antibacterial agents that inhibit the bacteria that cause acne. It also helps treat slow-healing wounds such as eczema and burns.

For normal skin types, mash the flesh of half a medium-sized organic avocado into a creamy texture. Massage into the face and neck, leave on for 15–20 minutes. Gently rinse off with warm water, then, if you wish, dab your skin with cool green tea.

For very dry and mature skin types, add 1 tablespoon of manuka honey to the mashed avocado.

If your skin is oily, add 1 teaspoon of freshly squeezed organic lemon juice and 1 tablespoon of manuka honey to the mashed avocado. Use the same day.

DID YOU KNOW? **UNIQUE MANUKA FACTOR (UMF)**

This is the rating used to indicate levels of antibacterial properties in active manuka honey. The Honey Research Unit at New Zealand's Waikato University indicates levels of 10+ as having special uses. The UMF makes it effective even against notorious 'super bugs' – strains of bacteria resistant to antibiotics.

nourishing banana mask

This face mask will gently detoxify and rehydrate your skin, leaving it glowing. Bananas are a good source of potassium, vitamins A, B6 and C are wonderfully effective at softening and hydrating the skin. Our skin has a protective layer to keep water in and foreign substances out. Cold or hot weather, wind, air-conditioning and heating can all damage this layer, making it dry and flaky. When you smear this banana mixture on your face, oil molecules form a temporary waterproof layer over your face, giving your skin cells a chance to rebuild their moisture levels.

Mash together half a small organic banana, 1 teaspoon of hemp oil and 1 teaspoon of manuka honey. Smooth the mixture over your skin and leave for 10 minutes before gently rinsing it off with warm water. This mask won't keep so make it fresh whenever you want to use it.

green tea soothing spray

Green tea (*Camellia sinensis*) is a powerful antioxidant and inhibits bacterial growth. The leaves contain tannic acid which is cooling on the skin (especially for sunburn). It also contains catechins, which help prevent and can even repair skin damage.

Steep 1 cup of organic green tea leaves in 1 litre of boiling, filtered water for 20 minutes. Cool and strain the liquid into a sterilised bottle and refrigerate. It will keep for eight days. If your skin is prone to blemishes add 1 teaspoon of dried sage or basil before making the infusion.

In addition to making a refreshing facial mist or blemish remedy – splash on, do not rinse – this infusion can be used to freshen strained or tired eyes. Soak cotton pads in green tea solution, squeeze out excess, and lay gently on closed eyelids. Leave for 10 minutes. Repeat if necessary. It can also be used as a perk-up for tired feet or an anti-fungal foot soak, or to soothe minor sunburn: soak a cloth in the tea and place on the sunburned area for about 15 minutes.

" For thousands of years women have turned to nature to help enhance their own beauty. The ancient Romans used beauty packs consisting of raw eggs mixed with honey. "

oatmeal and banana exfoliator

Oatmeal is highly absorbant, hypoallergenic and helps soften skin and heal dry, itchy skin. Of all the cereal grains, oats have the best balance of amino acids, which work as water-binding agents in skin care products.

If you have oily or acne-prone skin, add 1 tablespoon of organic fine oatmeal to the banana mask mix (see page 135). The small grains will gently exfoliate your face, removing dead skin and trapped dirt.

pineapple or papaya exfoliator

Pineapple contains the natural enzyme bromelain, which helps to break down the keratin proteins that form dead skin cells and so has a natural exfoliating effect that helps to improve skin texture. Papaya is rich in the natural enzyme papain, which also has skin-smoothing properties.

Simply rub a thin slice of pineapple or papaya over your skin to lift dead skin cells and exfoliate the skin. Leave to act for five minutes then rinse off with tepid water.

keeping your sparkle

Modern life puts a lot of stress on our eyes. Tiredness, dust, smoke, makeup, UV-radiation and bright computer screens all contribute to the problem. The skin around the eye is very thin, and so also very sensitive. It has few oil glands and little elasticity. It also contains many blood vessels that are easily visible. This may be why slow blood flow and a build-up of lymph causes dark 'circles' or shadows under the eyes and may also account for puffy eyes or the 'morning after' look. It is important to look after your eyes by following simple, healthy lifestyle measures.

● ●

EYE CARE TIP **TAKE REGULAR SCREEN BREAKS**

Peering at a computer screen all day long can lead to discomfort. In part, this is because we blink about 25 per cent less than normal when working at a computer, which causes eye dryness. To help keep your eyes well moistened, regularly close your eyes and count to five before opening them again. Regularly look away from the screen and focus on a faraway object, such as a building or tree on the skyline. If you get into this habit, your eyes should feel much less tired at the end of your working day.

● ●

keep them protected

UV-rays can cause serious damage to your eyes so always wear
sunglasses with UV filter in bright sunshine and make sure they
block at least 98 per cent of UV radiation. In the summer, you
need to wear sunglasses on overcast days as well, as clouds are no
barrier to UV light. Wear sunglasses even if your contact lenses
offer UV protection. Even high quality lenses only protect the area
they cover, but the entire surface of the eye needs protection.
Wearing sunglasses is especially important when reading out of
doors, as white paper reflects 80 per cent of the sun's rays.

eat well for healthy eyes

Antioxidants help prevent, or slow down, age-related eye
conditions such as macular degeneration and cataracts. Vitamins
C, A and E, folic acid, minerals selenium and zinc and especially
beta-carotene are highly beneficial for the health of your eyes.
Add carrot sticks and a bunch of grapes to your lunch box.

keep well lit

Make sure there is sufficient ambient light, especially when you
are reading or using a computer. Working in poor light causes
eyestrain, while very bright light can be just as harmful. Where
possible, work in natural light but seek shade from direct sunlight.
When working at the computer turn down the brightness on your
monitor and have a soft light coming from the side.

common eye problems

The most common eye problems arising from our modern lifestyle are dark circles under the eyes, puffiness and dry, irritated eyes. Here are some simple solutions:

dark circles

Over time, the skin of the eyelids gets thinner, making the underlying blood vessels more apparent and giving a darker appearance. Make sure you're getting 7–8 hours sleep a night and set aside some time just for yourself at least once a week to do something really relaxing. Dehydration can cause the skin under the eyes to look dark and puffy. Drink plenty of fluids and reduce your salt intake. Identify and treat any food allergies, which might contribute to the problem and make sure you are getting enough vitamins (see pages 58–9). Here are some more simple tips to lighten dark circles:

* Potatoes contain an enzyme called catecholase, which is used in some cosmetics as a skin lightener. Cut a round slice from a potato and cut in half to form two half-moons. Put one half-moon on the skin just under each eye and leave in place for 20 minutes.

* Make a poultice by soaking tea bags containing green tea in a little hot water. Allow the bags to cool until slightly warm then place over your closed eyes for 10–15 minutes.

* Dip cotton pads in rosewater, or cold milk. Lie down with your feet raised higher than your head then place the wet pads on your closed eyes. Relax for 10 minutes.
* Place hot and cold cloths alternately under the eyes for 10 minutes. Then apply some almond oil to the dark surface before going to bed.
* Press the acupressure point for eyes, located on the mound on your palm just below the index finger.

eye puffiness

Fluid is sometimes trapped in the tissues under the eyes, causing swelling or puffiness and itchy, red eyes, especially when you awake. Puffy eyes can be caused by changes in fluid balance, hormones, alcohol, weather or travel. They can also be hereditary. Puffy eyes can also be a sign of an allergy or dermatitis – especially if they're also itchy or red – or of sinus or even thyroid problems. Check with a medical practitioner to rule these out. Dry eyes could also indicate a lack of essential fatty acids (see pages 50–3).

Drinking plenty of water, herbal teas and diluted juices helps reduce eye puffiness. Make sure your bedroom is well ventilated – a hot environment will add to your puffy eye problem. Here are some more simple tips to reduce puffiness:

* Gently tap your skin with your ring finger when applying eye cream or gel to help excess fluid drain away. Puffy eyes respond well to products containing soothing herbal compounds such as azulene – found in blue chamomile oil.

141

- ✳ Store eye creams and gels in the fridge, as the cold helps reduce puffiness.
- ✳ Place strips of grated potato under your eyes to help reduce swelling. Strawberries and cucumber can help, too.
- ✳ Make a cup of green tea and allow to steep for five minutes or until cool. Wipe the eyes with this solution several times a day. Make fresh every day to avoid infection.
- ✳ Fill a small bowl with iced water. Soak a cotton wool pad with the liquid and lie down with the dampened pads over your eyes. Replace the pads as soon as they become warm. Continue for 15 minutes, replacing the pads as necessary.
- ✳ If your eyes are puffy in the morning, wrap an ice cube in a paper towel and hold it over each eyelid for a few minutes to reduce the swelling.

● ●

EYE CARE TIP **SOOTHE IRRITATED EYES**

If your eyes are red and itchy or inflamed, bathe them in a solution of eyebright herb (Euphrasia) – a teaspoon of eyebright in a cup of hot water. Make up two separate cups of this infusion – one for each eye – and use separate cotton balls for each eye. Steep the herb in the water for five minutes, until cool, strain and dip a cotton ball into the liquid and wipe your eye. Alternatively use cooled chamomile tea bags.

● ●

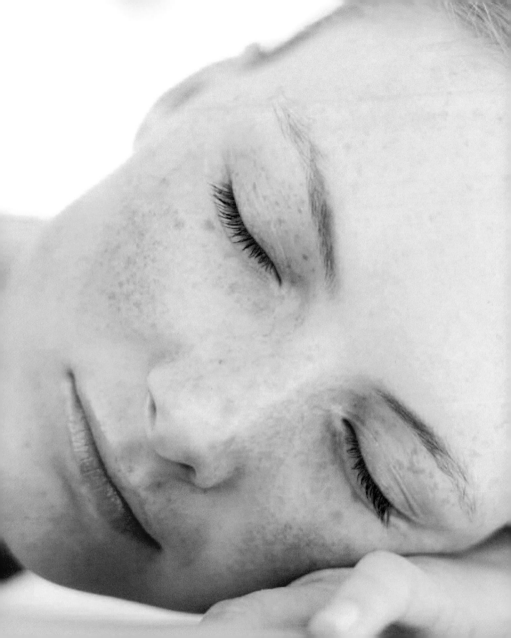

lovely lips

There is nothing like a beautiful smile to light up a face – it makes you look more attractive and lively. However, the lips are delicate and need extra care. Unlike the rest of the face, the lips are not skin as such but mucous membrane. This means they do not produce oil and lack protective melanin pigment. So it can be a challenge to keep them smooth and crack free. Lip problems are especially common in winter or in hot sunny weather.

Lips can also develop inflammation and cracks due to tiredness, depression, allergic reaction to cosmetics or toothpaste, skin infections, extreme weather conditions (for example if exposed to strong sunshine or wind), dehydration, habitual biting of the lips or vitamin B deficiency.

Wrinkles in the upper lips can be a sign of dehydration, so ensure you keep well hydrated inside and out, and quit smoking. Eat a well-balanced diet rich in fresh organic fruits and vegetables.

"Cold sores are caused by a virus – herpes simplex. The virus hides in the nerve root until activated and can be triggered by colds, menstrual periods, emotional upset, fatigue, bright sunlight and wind."

● ●

DID YOU KNOW? **FULL LIPS**

Your lips will look fuller and more sexually alluring when your oestrogen
levels are at their highest, just before ovulation.

● ●

caring for your lips

❋ Choose a non-petroleum based lipstick or lip balm made with
natural oils and waxes and UV-protection. Beeswax, carnauba
wax or berry wax protect the lips; base oils and essential oils
help to nourish and heal them.

❋ Gently massage a damp, soft-bristle toothbrush or washcloth
over your lips to smooth away rough spots. When the surface is
smooth, dry your lips with a clean towel.

❋ Apply a rich natural lip balm before bedtime.

❋ Avoid licking or biting your lips.

❋ Supplement your diet with vitamins B and C.

❋ Apply a moisturiser or lip balm before applying your lipstick –
choose an organic lipstick free from petrochemicals.

❋ If your lips are sore, try treating them with healing manuka
honey mixed with a little olive oil.

caring for your gums

One in three people over the age of 30 has some form of periodontal disease but is unaware of the problem because it develops silently and painlessly. Periodontal disease occurs when bacteria in plaque infect the gums and bones that anchor the teeth. Gum disease and dental decay are the primary causes of adult tooth loss. Bacterial toxins are then released into the bloodstream, beginning a cascade of health problems. Only your dentist can remove tartar build-up – you cannot brush tartar away.

brush and floss

It's not enough just to brush your teeth – even efficient brushing will remove only 60–70 per cent of plaque, the main cause of tooth decay and gum disease. To remove the remaining plaque you need to floss as well. The best time to floss is just before brushing your teeth. An electric toothbrush can remove plaque that resides just below the gum line. This will help you avoid gum disease.

effective mouthwashes

﹡ Add the juice of a freshly squeezed lemon to a glass of warm water and use as a mouthwash, holding it in the mouth for one minute. The lemon helps kill the bacteria that cause gingivitis, and the acid will dissolve plaque and strengthen the gums. – two remedies in one! Do this after every brushing. The tooth enamel will receive a coating from the toothpaste, which will protect it from the acidity of the lemon.

* Cranberries contain a compound that prevents bacteria from sticking to surfaces in the body. Rinsing the mouth with cranberry juice after meals could help to prevent the build-up of bacterial plaque. Use an unsweetened juice – sweetened ones are full of sugar, which will encourage bacterial growth!

* Both sage and sea salt have antiseptic properties that reduce inflammation and promote healing. They are also astringent, which helps tighten the gums. Pour a cup of boiling water over 1 tablespoon of sage leaves, cover and steep for 15 minutes, then strain add 2 teaspoons of sea salt. Use this mouthwash twice daily after brushing your teeth. Keep in the fridge and use within 3 days.

● ●

GUM-CARE TIP **USE AN SLS-FREE TOOTHPASTE**

More than 90 per cent of toothpastes currently on the market contain the foaming agent sodium lauryl sulphate (SLS). This harsh detergent is a persistent long-term irritant that is thought to cause tissue inflammation and increase the risk of gum disease (see page 189). Either use a detergent-free toothpaste or choose one that uses a milder alternative such as betaine. This natural ingredient stimulates saliva production and has a mild foaming action to soothe dry tongue and gums.

● ●

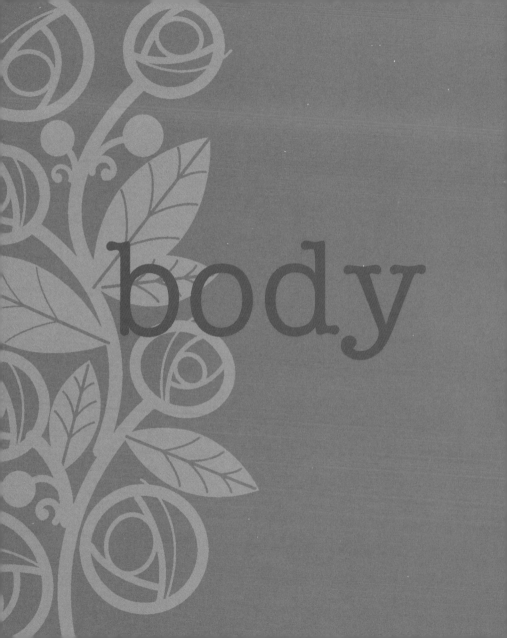
body

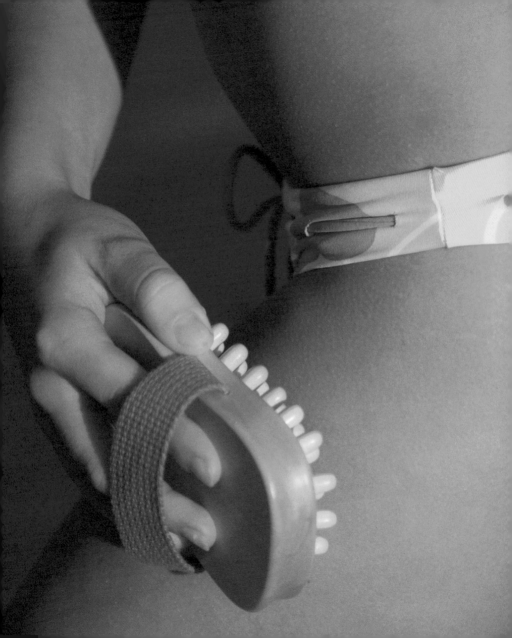

taking time for your body

It's all too easy to concentrate on facial skin care and neglect the rest of your body, especially your hands and feet. But all areas of the body need the same basic care that you lavish on your face, such as moisturising and exfoliating (see pages 154–5). And simple, natural treatments such as skin brushing and exfoliating are beneficial for your general health, too.

Pamper yourself!

I bet you can remember the last time you did a load of laundry, cooked, cleaned or went shopping, but when was the last time you took time out for you? Take the time to pamper yourself – everyone needs quality time for themselves.

Aim to spend a little time every day caring for your body, your hands and your feet. It doesn't matter if it is late evening or early morning – why not try waking up earlier than the others in the house to enjoy a few uninterrupted moments before the day fully begins? A few minutes set aside for yourself in this way will reap dividends for your skin and your sense of wellbeing.

> " If you have a demanding day ahead of you, take a nice long warm bath before you start. Fill your mind and senses with the fragrance of a pure essential oil and just soak for as long as you can. "

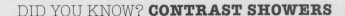

DID YOU KNOW? **CONTRAST SHOWERS**

A contrast shower – switching from hot to cold water – boosts the circulation, promotes detoxification and strengthens the immune system. It also helps to bring nutrients, oxygen and immune cells to damaged and stressed tissues, and carries away metabolic waste, inflammatory by-products and other toxic substances. Start with two to three minutes of hot (not scalding) water followed by less than one minute of cold water. Repeat once.

skin brushing

The skin covering your body is one of the most important organs for eliminating wastes, responsible for one-quarter of the body's detoxification. Lightly brushing your skin with a dry, natural brush stimulates blood and lymphatic circulation, removes dead skin cells and encourages new cell growth. Skin brushing brings nutrients and oxygen to the upper layer of skin. It also:

* tightens your skin
* improves digestion
* helps eliminate cellulite (see pages 156–9)
* increases cell renewal
* helps cleanse your lymphatic system
* removes dead skin cells
* strengthens your immune system

DID YOU KNOW? **THE LYMPHATIC SYSTEM**

The lymphatic system is a collection of tubes or lymph vessels running throughout the body that clears environmental toxins, wastes and infection from the tissues. Skin brushing stimulates the lymphatic system to help flush toxins from the body. The result is an improved ability to fight disease, and healthier and more resilient-looking skin.

" Most women with cellulite have a sluggish lymphatic system; getting this system flowing smoothly is the key to easy weight loss and improved feelings of wellbeing. "

tips for skin brushing

Skin brushing can be incorporated easily into a daily routine. It will take only two or three minutes, depending on how many strokes you give each area, yet the health benefits are tremendous!

❋ Brush your skin first thing in the morning, when the increased blood flow will help you wake up, or before a shower.

❋ Using a dry soft natural bristle brush, start at your feet and sweep up the legs in long, light, brisk movements.

❋ Don't be too rough: over brushing makes skin red and irritated.

❋ Brush from your fingertips up to your shoulders and towards the heart (to encourage the return of blood and encourage lymphatic flow). Use small strokes and gentle pressure.

❋ Avoid your face and any areas of skin irritation.

❋ Pay particular attention to cellulite-prone areas of your body such as the thighs.

❋ Brush your abdomen with a circular clock-wise motion.

❋ Make sure you wash your brush every few weeks in water and let it dry before using it again.

body exfoliation

Ready to invigorate and rejuvenate your skin? There is no better way than by using an exfoliating body scrub. Body scrubs regenerate your skin, help boost circulation, remove dead skin cells and open pores, allowing them to breathe. Exfoliating your skin once or twice a week is sufficient to:

✳ remove dead skin cells and surface toxins

✳ make the skin softer, smoother, fresher and brighter

✳ boost circulation and help unclog pores

✳ accelerate the growth of new cells

✳ give more even tanning

✳ allow new cells to absorb moisture applied to the surface

Caution: Skin exfoliation is not recommended for irritated or broken skin such as sunburn, rash or skin sores. To avoid skin irritation do not use a salt scrub after shaving.

● ●

BODY CARE TIP
EXFOLIATE BEFORE SELF-TANNING

Always exfoliate before you apply a self-tan lotion (see pages 214–17), taking care to remove every bit of dead skin or you will notice darker patches. Pay particular attention to your knees, elbows, feet and knuckles.

● ●

how to exfoliate

Start with a body brush (see pages 152–3) then take a bath or
shower so you are wet all over. Apply exfoliant scrub/cleanser to
your wash cloth (mild exfoliation) or loofah (extensive exfoliation).
Choose an exfoliator that contains natural ingredients such as
organic raw cane sugar, oatmeal, finely ground almonds,
pomegranate or cranberry. Body scrubs containing sugar crystals
are kinder to the skin than salt. The deep cleansing action of sugar
crystals is achieved without the drying effects often experienced
with salt-based products. Massage the exfoliator lightly but firmly
onto your body until a rosy glow appears. The massage action
improves circulation, breaking up fatty deposits that can cause
cellulite (see page 156). Rinse with warm water and towel dry.

exfoliating dry skin

As exfoliation strips off some of the skin's surface oils, choose an
oil-based sugar scrub if you suffer from dry skin and then massage
body oil into damp skin (after a bath or shower). If you have extra
thirsty skin, follow with a hydrating body lotion. This is a perfect
time to apply your cellulite lotion!

solutions for cellulite

Everyone has fat cells under their skin, whether they are old or young, curvaceous or slim. Cellulite occurs when fat cells become imprisoned in collagen and elastin fibres. As a result, circulation is slowed and nerve endings may become compressed and tender. Cellulite is most usually found on the buttocks, hips, and thighs, and sometimes on the back of the arms.

Hormones are primarily responsible for regulating fat storage and metabolism in the subcutaneous fat layer. In the late stages of pregnancy, oestrogens pull collagen tissue fibres apart, a crucial step in relaxing the cervix for childbirth. Therefore cellulite can appear during periods of hormonal change such as puberty, pregnancy, menopause, during the menstrual cycle and when using hormonal contraception for the first time. The following may also be responsible for cellulite:

* food allergies
* poor blood circulation
* lack of exercise
* eating the wrong types of foods
* dieting
* poor lymphatic system drainage (see page 152)

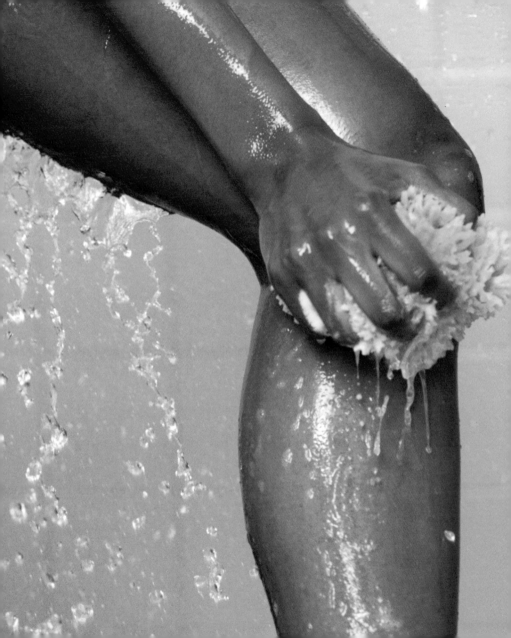

● ●

DID YOU KNOW? **CELLULITE AND OBESITY**

Although cellulite may look more prominent on overweight individuals, you can actually have as little as 14 per cent body fat and still have cellulite.

● ●

how to get rid of cellulite

To fight cellulite, you need to strengthen and hydrate the cells and connective tissue in your body. The following will help:

❊ Brush your skin every day (see pages 152–3).

❊ Improve your diet (see below).

❊ Exercise regularly to stimulate your circulation.

❊ Apply a cellulite lotion with scientifically proven
  active ingredients.

cleansing diet

A healthy eating plan will help to improve your inner health, in particular functions such as blood circulation and lymph flow.

❊ Start the day with a glass of warm water with a squeeze of
  lemon to stimulate digestion and revitalise the body.

❊ Add lots of fresh, organic fruit to your diet.

❊ Drink plenty of water and non-diuretic herbal teas.

❊ Avoid junk food, processed food and saturated fats.

❊ Include essential fatty acids in your diet.

exercise to combat cellulite

Cellulite-prone parts of your body, such as the buttock and thighs,
are prime areas for exercise. Try strength training; it increases
muscle tone and decreases total body fat. Leg curls and squats
with light weights are great for toning the thighs and buttocks.
Don't use weights that are too heavy – toning is the goal, not
muscle-building! Exercise with light weights three times a week.
Your weight-lifting exercise schedule can be as little as 15 minutes
three days a week. Circuit training is good because it fatigues the
muscle groups, helping to promote a reduction in the actual size of
the area, while decreasing the percentage of body fat.

● ● ● ● ● ● ● ● ● ● ● ● ● ● ● ● ● ● ●

DID YOU KNOW? **CELLULITE LOTIONS**

Traditional cellulite products use caffeine, or a caffeine equivalent, to
dehydrate the skin. This gives only a temporary tightening effect, as the
body is constantly rehydrating the skin. The newer cellulite lotions stop the
body storing excess fatty tissue and strengthen the skin surface. The results
last significantly longer than caffeine-based products.

● ● ● ● ● ● ● ● ● ● ● ● ● ● ● ● ● ● ●

treating skin disorders

The most common skin disorders affecting the body are forms of dermatitis, and psoriasis. Dermatitis is a broad term that covers a range of inflammatory skin disorders, including eczema.

Eczema leads to dry, itching and inflamed skin, sometimes with itchy blisters. The skin is highly sensitive, especially to cosmetics, soaps and harsh detergents. The severity of the condition ranges from a few dry, red, itchy patches to large areas of the body becoming covered in sore, inflamed, weeping and bleeding skin, which is easily infected.

ATOPIC ECZEMA

Atopic eczema is the commonest form of eczema and is closely linked with asthma and hay fever. It affects all ages and often runs in families. Symptoms of atopic eczema include dry, almost unbearably itchy and inflamed skin. Constant scratching can cause open wounds that are prone to infection. If eczema becomes infected the skin may crack and weep – a condition that is known as 'wet' eczema.

Dust mites, a common cause of atopic eczema, thrive in warm, moist environments such as bedding, mattresses, curtains and carpets. To prevent dust mites, air bedding well, avoid carpets in the bedroom, use a powerful vacuum cleaner and dust with damp micro-fibre cloths.

skin care for atopic eczema

❋ Avoid harsh soaps, shower gels, shampoos and bath products, especially those containing sodium lauryl sulphate (see page 189) and petrol-based ingredients such as petrolatum and paraffin wax, which stop the skin breathing. Products containing alcohol (ethanol) dry the skin and can make it sting and itch.

❋ Instead, use emollients such as hemp seed oil (see page 162) to keep the skin moist. Base oils vary and not all will be suited for your skin type (see pages 130–1). If in doubt, ask for a sample before you purchase.

❋ Avoid products containing harsh preservatives and synthetic fragrances. Even essential oils can be a problem for some eczema sufferers.

❋ To reduce the itching, choose cotton clothing and bedding to keep the skin cool and allow it to breathe. Avoid synthetic fabrics and wool, which can irritate.

❋ Use a gentle washing powder and avoid fabric softeners.

❋ At night, cotton mittens help reduce the damage that children can cause to their skin by scratching in their sleep.

❋ Stress can make eczema worse, so try to manage stress and practise relaxation techniques (see pages 16–17).

" Eczema is a highly individual condition so it is difficult to find a cure-all. A qualified kinesiologist will often be able to identify the 'hostile' substance or substances you are reacting to. "

● ●

DID YOU KNOW? **HEMP SEED OIL**

Hemp seed oil is made up of 80 per cent essential fatty acids and contains the ideal ration of omega-3 and -6. It does not just coat the skin, as most other oils do, but also nourishes deep skin tissue and prevents moisture loss. It offers relief for eczema, acne, psoriasis and minor abrasions.

● ●

diet for atopic eczema

❋ Supplements of zinc, and the B-vitamin biotin may be helpful.

❋ Increase your intake of omega-3 fatty acids.

❋ Eat lots of fresh vegetables and start juicing (see page 46).

❋ For adults, a detox diet (see pages 38–43) may help, too.

❋ Probiotics are especially beneficial in infant eczema.

❋ Take vitamin C to reduce histamine levels. (Eczema sufferers often produce high levels of this inflammatory chemical.)

❋ As a general rule, avoid dairy foods, especially cow's milk and cheese. Goat's milk is often better tolerated than cow's milk.

❋ Avoid foods containing wheat and yeast, fried and processed foods and refined sugar. Eggs, peanuts, tomatoes and citrus fruits – including fruit juices – can also trigger eczema.

❋ Atopic eczema can also be triggered by sensitivity to food ingredients and additives such as salicylate, amines, lactose, gluten, monosodium glutamate and sulphite preservatives.

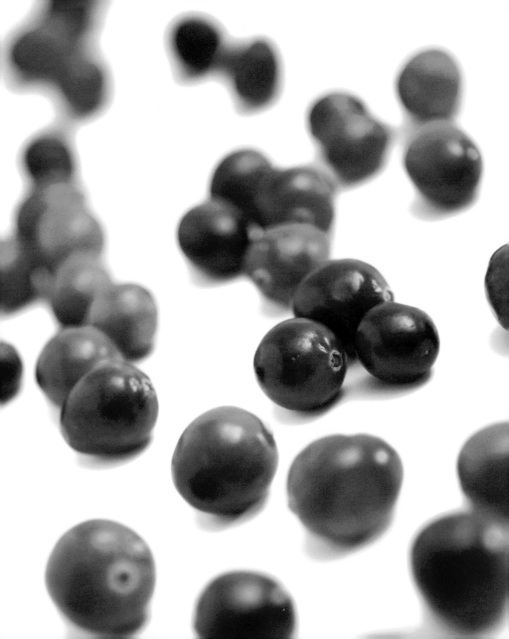

CONTACT DERMATITIS

There are two types of contact dermatitis: allergic contact
dermatitis and irritant contact dermatitis.

allergic contact dermatitis

This type of dermatitis usually develops over a long period of time
through regular contact with substances such as perfume, skin
care products, makeup and metals containing nickel. The best
form of prevention is to identify the cause of the rash and avoid it.

● ●

BODY CARE TIP **PREVENTING NICKEL ALLERGY**

To prevent allergic skin reactions to nickel, apply a thin coating of clear nail
varnish to the surface of metal in jewellery, watchstraps and studs on jeans.

● ●

irritant contact dermatitis

Contact with irritants such as household cleaners is the usual
cause of this form of dermatitis, which more usually affects adults.
As with the allergic form, the best prevention is to avoid contact
with the problem chemical. Always wear rubber gloves when
handling chemical cleaners and household detergents, or better
still clean your home with a micro-fibre cloth, hot water and organic
soap. Keep your hands well moisturised with organic hand lotion.

SEBORRHOEIC DERMATITIS

This can affect babies and adults. In babies it is often known as cradle-cap and can affect the scalp and nappy areas and quickly spread to the face, neck and armpits. It is not usually sore or itchy. In adults it looks very much like dandruff and can spread from the scalp to the face where flakes of skin can be shed from the eyebrows. This type of eczema is more common in men than in women and is often associated with a fungal infection. Seborrhoeic dermatitis usually clears after a few months but natural salves and bath oils can speed up the process. Products containing hemp oil and calendula are ideal.

● ●

DID YOU KNOW? **URINE THERAPY**

Urine therapy involves the use of one's own urine, taken internally or applied externally, to heal damaged skin or alleviate disease. Supporters of this therapy claim that it is effective for a wide range of conditions including colitis, lupus, rheumatoid arthritis, hyperactivity, psoriasis, eczema, herpes and adrenal failure. Fresh urine is sterile and consists of 95 per cent water. The remaining five per cent is made up of a mixture of urea, vitamins, minerals, enzymes, hormones, proteins and antibodies. Advocates argue that it is these substances that give urine its medicinal powers.

● ●

PSORIASIS

Psoriasis is characterised by raised circular plaques or patches of white or pink flaky skin, especially on the elbows, knees and scalp, although it can affect any part of the body. The exact cause is unknown but it is thought that in psoriasis new skin cells are produced many times faster than normal, resulting in a build-up of thick scales of dead skin. This may be an auto-immune response, possibly following bacterial or viral infection, or due to environmental or other factors. Flare-ups can be aggravated or triggered by medication, excess alcohol, obesity, too much or too little sunlight, poor health, injury, trauma, stress, cold and damp.

Treatment regimes that work well for one person may not help another, but some basic self-heal tips are beneficial for most people. It is generally accepted that there is a link between psoriasis and the nervous system, and managing stress levels, for example by learning some good relaxation techniques and getting a good night's sleep, will usually help. Using only natural fibres such as cotton and silk clothing and bed linen will help to reduce irritation. Psoriasis is often improved by moderate exposure to sunlight. Apply moisturiser before using a sun lotion. Some sunscreens aggravate itching and flaking, so choose natural, organic lotions and avoid the sun when it is at its strongest (between 11am and 3pm).

" Psoriasis is derived from the Greek word 'psor', which means itch. Around two per cent of the population have psoriasis to a greater or lesser degree. Psoriasis is not contagious. "

diet and psoriasis

Foods suspected of aggravating psoriasis include animal fats, acids, spices, salt and stimulants such as alcohol, tea, coffee and soft drinks. Increasing your intake of essential fatty acids can often help (see pages 50–3). Another cause may be overgrowth of the fungal infection *Candida albicans*. Removing sugars, refined starches, alcohol and yeast-based foods from the diet is worth exploring.

Psoriasis has been linked with consumption of acid-forming foods (see pages 32–7) and the recirculation of toxins from the intestinal tract. A switch to a more alkaline diet and detoxifying your intestines can aid the absorption of nutrients, enhance immunity and improve health.

Cleansing the colon, for example with high colonic irrigation, changing to a diet based on cleansing foods and supplementing with probiotics, has shown remarkable results for many psoriasis sufferers. Combining this with a high-fibre diet helps eliminate intestinal toxins and provides an environment that allows beneficial probiotic bacteria to thrive.

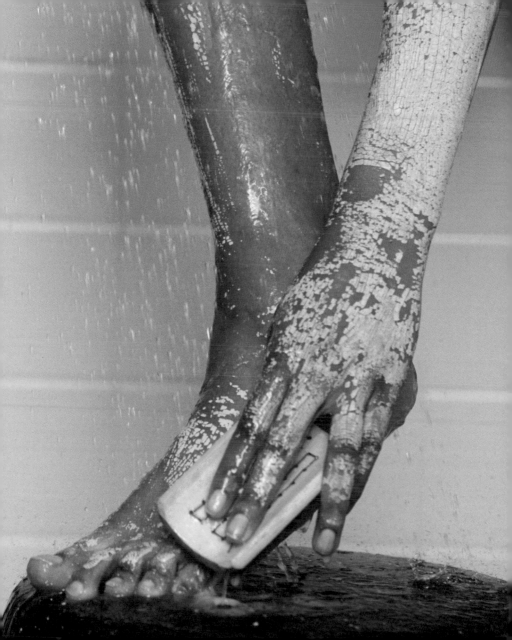

skin care for psoriasis

* Avoid harsh household products, biological washing powders, fabric conditioners, foaming agents such as sodium lauryl sulphate and products containing perfume and colouring.

* If you suffer from psoriasis of the scalp, take your own brand of gentle shampoo and conditioner when you visit the hairdressers to avoid irritation from branded products. Shampoos containing bromelain, an enzyme found in pineapple, can reduce inflammation and calm the immune response.

* Use only gentle, natural skin care products. Look for those containing chickweed, to help relieve itching, hemp oil (see page 79), to moisturise and soothe irritation, chamomile and calendula, for their anti-inflammatory and healing action, and the skin-soothing herb marshmallow.

* Apply your natural skin salve, moisturiser or body butter before bathing to soothe and moisturise your skin.

* Treat yourself to an Epsom salt or Dead Sea salt bath. Dead Sea mud can also be used as a body treatment.

healthy hands

The hands work harder than any other part of the body and, despite having fewer sebaceous glands than the rest of the body, they are frequently exposed to heat, cold, UV light, water and chemicals. Little wonder that the first signs of ageing often show on your hands. A good hand care regime is vital to keep your hands healthy and looking good.

daily care

* Dry skin not only looks wrinkled but is also easily damaged.
* Ensure that your hands are properly dried after being in water or – ironically – the skin will quickly dry out.
* Moisturise your hands several times a day.
* Improve circulation and release tension by stretching or bending your fingers for a few seconds several times a day.
* Protect your hands by wearing rubber gloves when washing up, cleaning and gardening.
* Use SPF 15 sun lotion when outdoors.

weekly care

Each week, give your hands a gentle sugar scrub massage. Rub your hands with a small amount of sugar scrub, massage gently for one minute and rinse thoroughly with warm water. Wipe excess oils away with a paper towel and pat dry.

Alternatively make your own hand exfoliator. Add 2 tablespoons of organic olive oil to 3 tablespoons of granulated sugar. Mix to a paste and follow the instructions above.

skin care for dry hands

* Mix 1 tablespoon of organic honey with 2 tablespoons of organic unsalted butter. Apply the mixture to clean hands and massage in well for a couple of minutes. Wipe off excess any with a hand towel.
* Mashed potatoes with milk (cow's or soya) makes a great hand mask. Massage it into your hands, leave for 2–3 minutes, then rinse and dry your hands.
* To restore the skin's pH balance, wash your hands in an organic apple cider vinegar solution (1 tablespoon of vinegar to 200ml water).

keeping your hands clean

Having dirty hands is one of the fastest ways to get and spread germs. But just washing your hands isn't enough – wet hands carry far more germs, so remember to dry them well. If you are particularly concerned about the spread of bacteria, look for liquid soaps that contain extracts of tea tree and manuka. Both these ingredients have powerful antibiotic properties, but unlike some anti-microbial agents (see below), they do not carry the risk of causing bacterial resistance to antibiotics or harm the environment.

● ●

DID YOU KNOW? **TRICLOSAN**

Many hand washes contain powerful anti-microbial agents such as triclosan. However there are concerns that their widespread use could be contributing to the increase in antibiotic-resistant bacteria such as MRSA. There are also fears that triclosan reacts with chlorine in tap water to produce highly toxic dioxins, which can interfere with hormone production. Finally, because triclosan residues in waste water are extremely toxic to algae – the basis of the aquatic food chain – there are concerns about long-term environmental effects. Triclosan is present in many other personal care products, too, including soaps, mouthwashes, toothbrushes, cosmetics, deodorants, shaving gel and creams, and is also increasingly being added to a range of children's toys, clothing and household products, usually under the name of MicrobanTM.

● ●

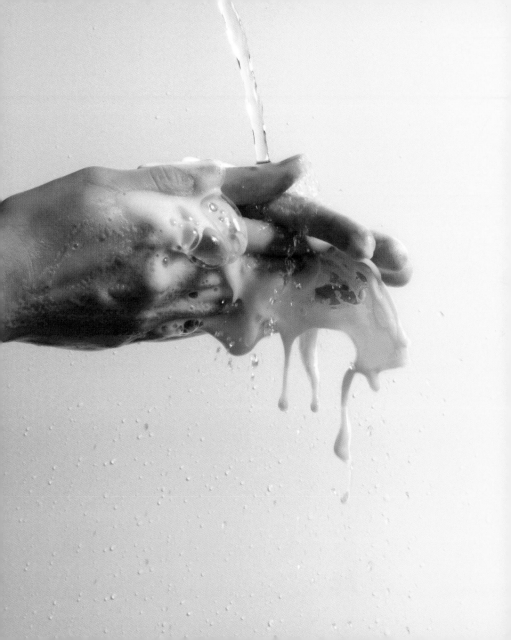

NAILS

Nails soon show signs of stress, illness and poor diet. Nails grow at around 1mm per week but growth soon slows down if you have any nutrient deficiency. Common signs of nutrient deficiency are:

* **White spots or flecks** usually indicate a zinc deficiency. Sometimes also caused by taking the contraceptive pill.
* **Ridged or brittle nails** can be a sign of vitamin A and calcium deficiency.
* **Cuts and cracks in the nails** may indicate that you need to drink more fluids.
* **Splitting nails** could indicate insufficient hydrochloric acid production or a lack of essential fatty acids in your diet.
* **Dryness and very rounded and curved ends** may be caused by insufficient intake of vitamin B12 or be the result of an iron deficiency.

nail care tips

* To remove dirt and stains, mix 1 tablespoon of lemon juice in a cup of water. Soak the nails in the liquid and massage around the cuticles for a few minutes.
* To harden soft nails, soak your nails in warm organic olive oil for 20 minutes every other day.

diet for the nails

✳ Make sure that at least half your diet is based around fresh fruit and raw vegetables in order to supply necessary vitamins, minerals and enzymes.

✳ Eat foods rich in sulphur and silicon, such as broccoli, fish and onions, and include foods rich in biotin such as soya, brewer's yeast and whole grains.

✳ Supplement your diet with nutrient-rich wild seaweed (kelp).

●　●

DID YOU KNOW? **WILD SEAWEED (KELP)**

Wild seaweed contains more vitamins and minerals in its roots, stem and leaves than any other food. In particular it is rich in iodine, potassium, magnesium, calcium and iron, as well as many trace minerals. This spectrum of minerals supports the metabolism of all-important essential fatty acids and improves blood circulation in the skin. Iodine is vital for a healthy thyroid gland, which governs healthy hair, nails, skin and teeth.

●　●

happy feet

When it comes to beauty care, the one area of the body we take for granted is the feet. Yet they not only support us physically, they are also important on an emotional level as they represent our foundation, security and inner strength and our connection with the earth. All it takes is an irritation on a little toe to disturb your total wellbeing. Giving your feet a little consideration and loving care can make all the difference.

" If you often wear uncomfortable shoes, the odds are that at one time or another you will experience painful heels. By regularly stretching your Achilles tendon you can help relieve heel pain. "

shoes

A foot has up to 250,000 sweat glands, and your shoes can absorb up to 60 per cent of the moisture released each day. So alternate your shoes to allow them to air and dry out between wearing. Avoid buying shoes in the morning, as the feet expand during the day. When trying on shoes, wriggle your toes to make sure they are roomy enough. Shoes should be comfortable, and easy to put on at the time of purchase. Never expect them to 'break in'.

● ●

FOOT CARE TIP **EXERCISE FEET AND ANKLES**

Place 12 marbles on the floor. With bare feet, pick them up one by one with your toes and drop them into a plastic cup or bowl. Flex your ankles back and forth and practise clockwise and counter clockwise rotations several times daily to strengthen your feet and ankles.

● ●

pampering foot care routine

Follow this foot routine a few times a week and you will have lovely looking feet.

※ Remove the hard skin from your feet using a pumice stone or diamond dust file.

※ Apply cream generously to the area to remove dead skin.

※ Soak your feet in a bowl of warm water for about 10 minutes to soften the skin (add half a cup of Epsom salts or 5 drops of essential oil of your choice).

※ Dry your feet thoroughly, especially between your toes.

※ Massage your feet with rich foot skin cream. Cup your hands on either side of your foot and with your thumbs firmly press the upper part of your foot while pushing your thumbs outwards.

※ Gently massage the ankle bones in a circular motion to remove any stiffness in the ankle.

tired feet

Try these treats to soothe tired feet:

* After being on your feet all day, soak your feet in a bowl of warm water enriched with essential oils or Epsom salts – don't forget to moisturise your feet afterwards.

* Place a layer of glass marbles in the bottom of a large foot bowl – enough to cover about three-quarters of the base. Add just enough warm water to cover the feet, and add half a cup of Epsom salts and 3 drops of your favourite essential oil. Place your feet in the bowl and gently glide your feet along the marbles for a soothing massage. Soak for 10 minutes.

* A cooling, refreshing peppermint and eucalyptus foot bath will do wonders for tired or hot feet. Add 5 drops of essential oil to warm water and soak your feet for 10 minutes.

* For chronically cold feet, try a warming ginger foot bath. Add 1–2 teaspoons of fresh shredded ginger or 5 drops of ginger essential oil to a bowl of warm water and soak your feet for 10–20 minutes. Rinse and dry.

● ●

DID YOU KNOW? **EPSOM SALTS**

A solution of Epsom salts (magnesium sulphate) in water draws toxins from
the body, sedates the nervous system, reduces swellings and relaxes muscles.
It is a natural emollient and exfoliator, too. You can soak in Epsom salts to
soften skin or use them as a scrub to exfoliate rough patches. Epsom salts can
help reduce swelling and inflammation and are great as a skin stress reducer.

● ●

TREATING PROBLEM FEET

smelly feet

* Organic apple cider vinegar works well as an antifungal agent
  and deodoriser. Add half a cup to a bowl of warm water and
  soak your feet for 5–10 minutes.
* Alternatively try half a cup of deodorising baking soda.
* Buy a natural deodorising foot lotion and apply every morning
  after washing your feet.
* Spray your shoes with a solution of deodorising ammonium
  alum or alunite.

athlete's foot

Athlete's foot is commonly contracted at public swimming pools, showers and changing rooms. It will be aggravated if your feet sweat a lot or if you wear tight, non-breathable shoes or synthetic fibres next to the skin. It can also be a symptom of yeast overgrowth in the body. Avoid sugar, fruit juice, alcohol and yeasted breads, which may contribute to this condition.

Take a probiotic supplement and try an antifungal foot soak. Mix half a cup of organic apple cider vinegar with 5 drops of tea tree or manuka oil (both excellent anti-fungal agents) and 5 drops of lavender oil and add to a bowl of warm water. Soak your feet for 10 minutes. Dry thoroughly, especially between each toe, and apply some tea tree or manuka essential oil to the affected area.

● ●

DID YOU KNOW? **REFLEXOLOGY**

Reflexology is not only a treat for the feet, it can also alleviate problems in other parts of the body. Reflexologists believe that each area of the soles of the feet and toes corresponds to a specific body organ or area. Disorders or imbalances in the colon or kidneys, for example, will be indicated by tenderness on the related part of the sole. By massaging and stimulating the affected areas of the feet, the corresponding part of the body is also stimulated and restored to normal functionality. For a list of qualified reflexologists in your area, contact the National Register of Reflexologists.

● ●

swollen feet

A certain amount of swelling in your feet is natural, especially in warm weather, when standing on your feet all day, if you take oral contraceptives or habitually cross your legs, or during late pregnancy.

❋ Check that you are not having too much salt in your diet, or suffering from an underlying illness. Swollen feet can also be a sign of heart, kidney and liver disorders as well as minor vascular disorders. In serious or long-term cases, see your doctor.

❋ To alleviate swelling, sit down, remove your shoes and socks, and elevate your feet and legs by resting your heels on a pillow placed on a chair or high stool. If possible, soak your feet in cool water first.

❋ Take more exercise to improve your cardiovascular system and circulation, which will reduce the tendency of your feet to swell.

dry, callused feet

Try this overnight treat and you'll wake up with smooth, soft feet:

❋ Wash and towel dry feet.

❋ Massage each foot thoroughly with sugar scrub (see page 155) using small circular motions, concentrating especially on any areas of hard skin such as the heels.

❋ Rinse with warm water.

❋ Apply a generous amount of body butter or a good foot cream.

❋ Slip on a pair of cotton socks before getting into bed.

hair

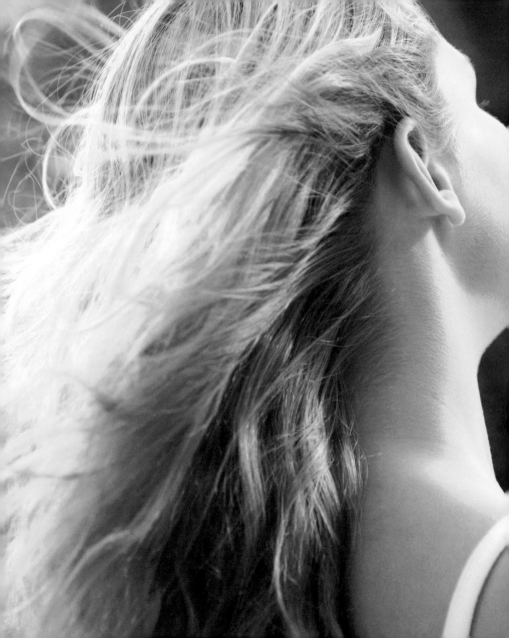

healthy hair

Hair is a barometer of your general health. Healthy hair comes with a healthy body. What goes into your body is reflected on the outside, including your hair. Hair needs adequate amounts of amino acids, vitamins A, B, C and E, minerals calcium, zinc, iron and copper and essential fatty acids. If the diet does not supply these nutrients (see pages 58–9), or the blood supply to the scalp is inadequate, the hair becomes dry or greasy, the ends split and it loses its bounce.

Alongside each hair lies a sebaceous gland (see page 64) that secretes sebum to lubricate and help protect the hair. If the sebaceous glands produce more sebum than needed, the hair becomes oily. If these glands are sluggish, hair becomes dry.

" Drinking plenty of water and eating lots of raw fruit and vegetables and sufficient protein is the best way to achieve healthy hair. "

keep it lubricated

For hair to be in tiptop condition it needs a moisture (water) content of at least 8 per cent, and the right balance of protein and natural oil (sebum). Most of us produce enough sebum to keep our hair healthy, but often lack moisture. Many hair care oils, unlike essential oils, cannot penetrate the hair shaft, but lie on the outside. With repeated applications, residue builds up preventing moisture penetrating and so the hair cannot be rehydrated. These oils do not diffuse or evaporate. If you use hot styling tools or spend time in very sunny climates, the problem is made worse.

keep it balanced

Just like the skin from which it grows, healthy hair is slightly acidic, with a pH around 5.5 (see pages 33 and 65). Alkaline hair care products upset the pH balance and produce a roughened surface leading to dry, rough, dull and frizzy hair. Even more distressing, weakened hair is brittle and easily damaged. Hair colourants, permanent waving solutions and heat treatments such as hair driers, rollers and ceramic hair straighteners also affect the pH and contribute to the damage. To protect your hair, use a pH balanced, natural shampoo and conditioner.

● ●

DID YOU KNOW? **KERATIN**

Hair is made of keratin, a strong, elastic protein also found in nails. The outer layers are the cuticle. Under a microscope, this looks like a tiled roof. When hair is in good condition the cuticle layers lie together, giving hair a smooth, shiny appearance. When hair is in poor condition, the cuticle layers lift, becoming uneven and easily damaged. Hair feels coarse and brittle and, as it can't reflect light, looks dull and lifeless.

● ●

hair care programme

A healthy head of hair requires an ongoing hair care routine. The following programme will keep your hair looking great.

washing

* Comb the tangles out of your hair before washing as wet hair is extremely fragile.
* Use a gentle shampoo to preserve the hair's acid coating.
* With any shampoo – even gentle, natural, organic types – rinse thoroughly to remove all traces of detergents from the hair roots. Detergents irritate the scalp and inhibit hair growth.
* Wash your brushes and combs regularly with shampoo.

● ●

HAIR CARE TIP **COMBAT CHLORINE**

Are your highlights turning green from exposure to chlorine in swimming pools? Simply grab the ketchup bottle and pour lots on your hair! Work it in carefully with your fingers or a wide toothed comb. Leave for at least 20 minutes then shampoo and rinse with cold water.

● ●

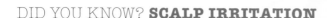

DID YOU KNOW? **SCALP IRRITATION**

Detergent residues are often the primary cause of scalp irritation, as well as of excessive sebum and hair loss.

conditioning and rinsing

✻ Use a small amount of conditioner on the hair, especially the ends (but avoid getting conditioner on the roots). Leave for 1–2 minutes and then comb through very gently and rinse well.

✻ If you have dark hair or a flaky, itchy scalp, rinse your hair with diluted organic cider vinegar (20ml vinegar in 200ml water).

✻ For fair hair and a greasy scalp, rinse with diluted juice of half a lemon in 200ml water.

✻ Now pat and squeeze your hair dry – do not rub.

blow-drying

✻ Wait until your hair is at least half dry before you style it.

✻ Dampen the dry ends with a herbal mist or foam to reduce heat damage.

✻ Dry your hair from roots to end – keeping the dryer at least 15–20cm away.

✻ Dry in the following order: back, sides, crown then front.

✻ Tip your head upside down to increase volume.

shampoo

The main ingredients used in the majority of shampoos are water (80 per cent), detergents (10–15 per cent), thickeners (under 5 per cent), fragrances and preservatives. We've become accustomed to highly foaming shampoos, but you don't need to generate lots of bubbles to clean hair effectively. The majority of high street shampoos rely on inexpensive, petrochemical-derived detergents such as sodium lauryl sulphate (see opposite). Harsh synthetic detergents remove natural oils along with dirt, and every time you wash your hair your skin absorbs some of these chemicals.

what to use

Choose a gentle, natural shampoo. Several brands offer ultra-mild, concentrated, biodegradable and natural formulas. Look for shampoos that contain natural humectants such as glycerine, honey or sugar solution. These all attract moisture and hold it in the hair and, together with your natural sebum, help to restore and maintain your hair's moisture at its optimum level. Be cautious of the detergents in your shampoo. Opt for natural cleansing agents derived from corn, coconut, palm and olive oils, such as decyl, lauryl or coco glucoside, coco betaine or extracts from yucca or quillaja bark.

what to avoid

Avoid brands heavily laced with the following chemicals (some
known carcinogens):

* artificial colours (especially from coal tar)
* formaldehyde, polyethylene glycol and DMDM hydantion
* polysorbates 60 and 80
* propylene glycol
* quaternium 15
* sodium lauryl sulphate (SLS) – see below
* synthetic fragrance
* triethanolamine (TEA)
* 2-bromo-2-nitropropane-1,3-diol

● ●

DID YOU KNOW? **SLS AND SLES**

Sodium lauryl sulphate (SLS) is widely used by cosmetic manufacturers
because it produces rich foam and is cheap to formulate. However, it is a
major irritant, it denatures proteins and can cause skin and eye damage. Its
chemical make-up means it easily penetrates the skin and enters the
bloodstream. A similar substance, sodium laureth sulphate (SLES) is less
irritating, but a suspected carcinogen – 1,4 Dioxane – is a by-product of its
manufacture. SLS and SLES are not allowed in products certified to
European Organic Standards.

● ●

relaxing scalp massage

Massaging the scalp and hair with warm oil infused with hair-friendly herbs is a great way to nourish the scalp. It also relaxes your mind and nervous system, promotes sound sleep and may help your memory too. For maximum enjoyment ask someone else to do it for you. A warm oil massage, once a week:

* conditions the scalp, helping to prevent flaking and dry scalp
* relaxes the scalp and neck muscles, helping to combat stress and enhance blood circulation, so aiding hair growth
* strengthens and nourishes the hair roots and shafts, strengthening existing hair and promoting new growth

" My favourite massage is Indian head massage – 'champi' – which involves shiatsu and acupressure techniques. It not only relaxes tense areas but also helps rebalance your energy flow. "

how to massage your scalp

Jojoba oil is an ideal base oil for a scalp massage. Choose essential oils suitable for your hair type (see page 203).

* Pour a little oil into a bowl. Place the bowl in hot water to warm the oil. The oil should be warm but comfortable to the touch.

* Using the pads of your fingers, work the oil into your scalp, using circular motions. Slow, deliberate movements are relaxing while steady but vigorous movement helps enhance energy and circulation. Apply the oil a little at a time to different parts of the scalp, parting your hair as needed. Work some oil along the length of your hair.
* Cover your entire scalp, all the way down the sides to your ears and at the back to your neck.
* Leave the oil on for at least 30–60 minutes, longer if you can.
* After your massage, dip a towel in hot water, wring it out and wrap it around your head.
* You can even leave the oil on overnight – place a thick towel over your pillow to protect your bed linen.
* Wash out with a gentle, natural shampoo.

● ●

DID YOU KNOW? **ORGASMATRON**

Orgasmatron massages the pressure points around your head and the back of your neck. The flexible prongs are made of copper, which acts as a conductor, tapping into the body' s unique electrical fields. The orgasmatron will find countless pressure points with no particular skill needed. (See page 218 for stockist.)

● ●

treating dry frizzy hair

Contrary to common belief, dry, frizzy hair lacks water, not oils. When hair curls it forces the cuticle (the outer layer) to lift, which makes it dry out more easily. Perming lotions, hair dyes and bleaches can reduce its moisture level to as low as two per cent, leading to split ends. If moisture level is not restored to its normal eight per cent, split ends will worsen, leading to hair breakage.

If you spend lots of time in the sun, you'll need to supply the extra nutrition and moisture your hair needs. Conditioners that contain ingredients such as rice and wheat proteins help to repair damaged cuticles and improve porosity and elasticity.

what to do

* Trim regularly (short hair every 6 weeks; long hair, 8–12 weeks).
* Follow a weekly conditioning treatment.
* Rinse your hair with a solution of baking soda to get rid of shampoo build-up and styling residues.
* Rinse your hair with lemon juice to bring back life and shine.
* Apply apple cider vinegar mixed with water to your hair to give it shine and bounce.
* Rub jojoba oil into your hands and apply sparingly to your hair.
* Add essential oil of ylang ylang to your shampoo, conditioner and styling agents as a hair rejuvenator. (Ylang ylang and rosemary essential oils also stimulate hair growth.)

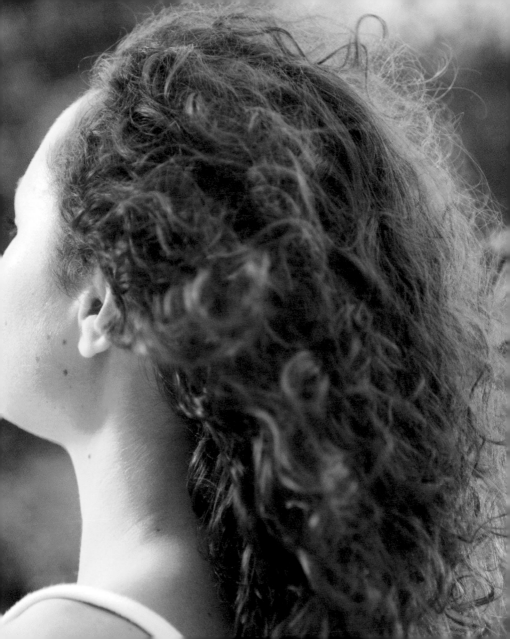

common scalp problems

Many hair problems occur when the scalp is under stress. Symptoms include itching and flaking (dandruff), dry scalp or persistent scalp irritation. Common causes are harsh styling procedures, hypersensitivity to food or personal care ingredients and psychological stress.

dry, flaky scalp

The most common cause of dry, flaking scalp is using shampoos containing harsh detergents such as SLS (see page 189). Other causes include over-shampooing, hair sprays containing alcohol, changes of climate and central heating.

❋ Try a simple conditioning mixture of rosemary essential oil and olive oil. Comb into wet, clean hair and wrap your head in a warm towel for 45 minutes, then use a mild shampoo.

❋ In winter, place a small humidifier in your bedroom at night.

itchy scalp

An itchy scalp often indicates an allergic reaction to an ingredient in your hair care product, usually a detergent or perfume. Rinsing with highly chlorinated water can also cause scalp irritation.

❋ Choose a mild, perfume-free shampoo.

❋ Rinse thoroughly after washing.

❋ Avoid any harsh styling products.

● ●

DID YOU KNOW? **SILICONE WAX IN SHAMPOO**

Most commercial shampoos contain silicone wax to smooth the hair,
but the wax residue often accumulates on your scalp. Perspiration beneath
the wax residue left behind is susceptible to bacterial growth. When you
scratch, the bacterial infection will cause your scalp to feel itchy.

● ●

dandruff

We all shed flakes of dead skin from the scalp every day, but some
people experience an unusually large amount of flaking and suffer
repeated outbreaks. Although dandruff is often considered a dry
skin condition, many sufferers have greasy hair and an oily scalp.
There may also be a link between dandruff and the skin fungus
Malassezi globosa.

* Regularly wash your hair with a mild, SLS-free shampoo to
  remove excess flakes. Use one containing bromelain, a plant
  enzyme that helps release skin flakes from the scalp.
* Massage the scalp with jojoba oil to help calm overactive
  sebaceous glands.
* Tea tree and manuka essential oils and extracts help control
  fungal growth often linked to dandruff. Add a few drops to
  your shampoo or mix with jojoba oil for a scalp massage.
* Increase your intake of essential fatty acids (see pages 50–3).

why hair thins as we age

We lose hair as each one comes to the end of its natural life – between two and seven years. The hair detaches from the follicle and, after a resting phase, a new hair grows in its place.

From your mid-20s onwards, the hair follicles and scalp receive less nourishment from the blood. This leads to a gradual decline as the hair becomes weaker, thinner, duller and more prone to damage. Poor diet and illness can contribute to the problem, and you can easily damage your hair with heating appliances, overuse of chemical treatments, and by washing your hair with harsh shampoos and not rinsing thoroughly. In addition, trauma, stress and anxiety reduce blood supply to the scalp, which contributes to temporary hair loss. Hair thinning can also be due to:

* hormonal changes, especially after the menopause
* medical conditions such as hypothyroidism
* medications including non-steroidal anti-inflammatory drugs (NSAIDs), such as aspirin; antibiotics, antidepressants, ulcer and heart medications and chemotherapy drugs
* intrinsic ageing
* malnutrition
* pregnancy
* genetic make-up
* over-brushing
* environmental factors – pollution, climate and seasonal changes

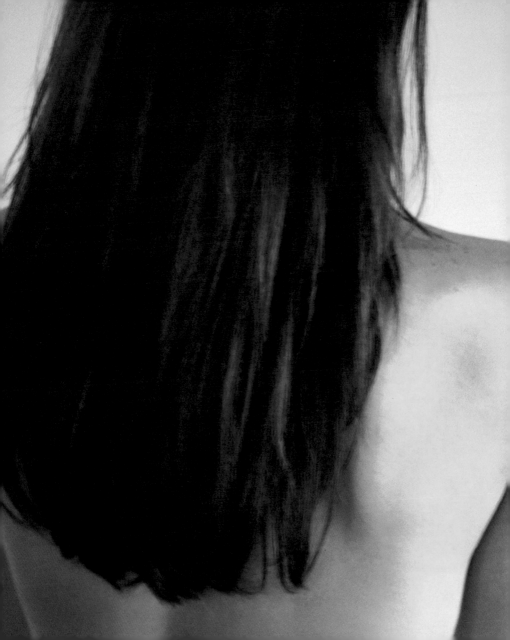

homemade hair treats

CONDITIONERS

conditioning pre-wash for dry hair

¼ cup organic olive oil

5 drops frankincense essential oil (other oils may be substituted if you wish)

Pour olive oil into a lidded container and add the essential oil. Place the lid on the container and shake well to disperse the essential oil. Leave to infuse for 24 hours in a cool, dark place. Shake again just before use.

Dampen your hair with warm water. Warm 1 tablespoon of the oil mix in the palms of your hands. Gently massage the oil into the entire scalp with your fingertips, using a circular motion. Rub the ends of your hair with the remaining oil. Place a shower cap, plastic bag or cling film over your hair. Cover plastic with a towel to retain body heat, which allows the oil to work better. Leave for at least 30 minutes. Rinse well, then shampoo and condition as usual.

"You can condition your hair from within by supplementing your diet with wild seaweed (kelp) capsules."

intensive pre-wash for thinning hair

100ml jojoba oil

15 drops rosemary oil

10 drops cedarwood oil

5 drops thyme oil

Mix the ingredients. Apply to your scalp and wrap in a hot towel
for at least 25 minutes. Rinse, then shampoo your hair as normal.

intensive conditioner for dry hair

1 egg yolk

150ml warm green tea

Whisk the egg yolk and then whisk the tea into it. Massage
throughout your hair, leave for 5 minutes and then rinse well with
lukewarm water (not hot or the egg will stick to your hair).

'degreaser' for oily hair

1 egg white

150ml warm green tea

Follow the instructions above.

conditioner for normal/dry hair

½ ripe avocado, mashed to a smooth paste

1 teaspoon avocado or olive oil

1 egg yolk

Blend all ingredients together and massage into your hair after
shampooing. Leave for 5 minutes, then rinse well.

HAIR RINSES

energising rinse

1 cup organic apple cider vinegar

1 cup spring water

10 drops rosemary essential oil

5 drops peppermint oil

Mix all the ingredients together. Shampoo and rinse your hair as usual then pour the energising rinse slowly over hair and work through from tips to roots.

" If your hair has lost its vitality, the problem could be due to product build-up. Give your hair a pampering treat with one of these hair rinses and your hair will soon regain its radiance. "

vitamin shine rinse

1 cup water

2 teaspoons organic cider vinegar

5 drops lemon essential oil

1 cup beer

5 drops rosemary essential oil

Mix all ingredients together. Shampoo and rinse your hair as usual, then pour the vitamin shine rinse slowly over the hair and work through to add softness and shine to your hair.

STYLING

hair gel

1 cup water

2 tablespoons flax seeds

1 tablespoon rosewater or similar

½ teaspoon glycerine

6 drops essential oil of your choice (see page 203)

Place the water and flax seeds in a small saucepan and bring to the boil. Remove from the heat and leave to infuse for 15 minutes. Strain out the seeds and allow to cool. Add the rosewater, glycerine and essential oil of your choice. This will keep for up to two weeks in the fridge.

hair spray

½ lemon, chopped

½ orange, chopped

2 cups water

4–6 drops essential oil of your choice (see page 203)

Place the chopped lemon and orange in a saucepan with the water and boil until reduced by half. Cool, strain and pour into a spray bottle. Add 4–6 drops of essential oil. This will keep for up to two weeks in the fridge.

essential oils for your hair

Essential oils can be extremely helpful in hair care as they influence the sebaceous glands and can normalise their functions. The oils penetrate deeply into the hair shaft and follicle and help produce healthy, shiny hair and encourage new hair growth. They can be used to:

* strengthen hair
* help control dandruff
* improve condition
* help an itchy, flaky scalp.

Some oils work directly on the hair, helping to restructure, repair or strengthen it. Other essential oils improve the condition of the hair by improving the condition of the scalp. Jojoba as well as almond, avocado and olive are great as base oils for scalp massage. Coconut oil should be used for hair treatments on dry, coarse hair.

" The scalp is a living organ – to have truly healthy-looking hair you must have a healthy scalp. Essential oils can work wonders on the condition of both your hair and scalp. "

hair type and essential oils

normal
Eucalyptus, cedarwood, geranium, orange, lavender, rosemary

oily
Basil, bergamot, cedarwood, cypress, grapefruit, lavender, lemon

dry
Frankincense, geranium, lavender, palmarosa, rosemary, sandalwood

damaged
Comfrey, horsetail, lavender, frankincense

fine
Geranium

dark
Rosemary, thyme

fair
Roman chamomile

grey
Sage

frequent wash
Geranium, horsetail, lavender, rosemary

thinning hair
Basil, clary sage, cypress, palmarosa, rosemary, thyme, cedarwood

dandruff
Cedarwood, rosemary, sage, tea tree, thyme, patchouli

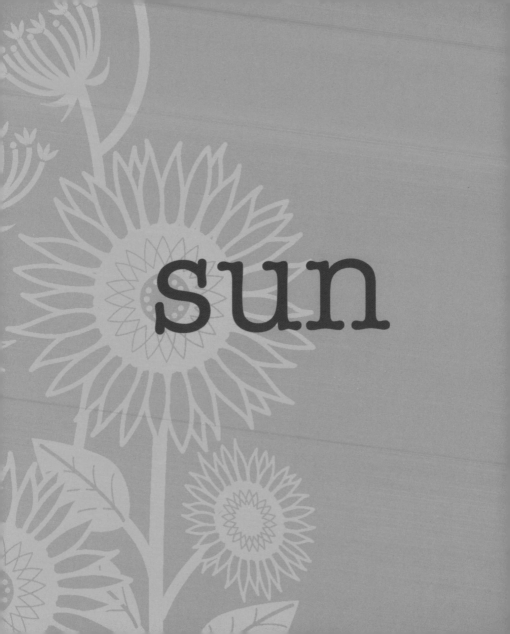

sun

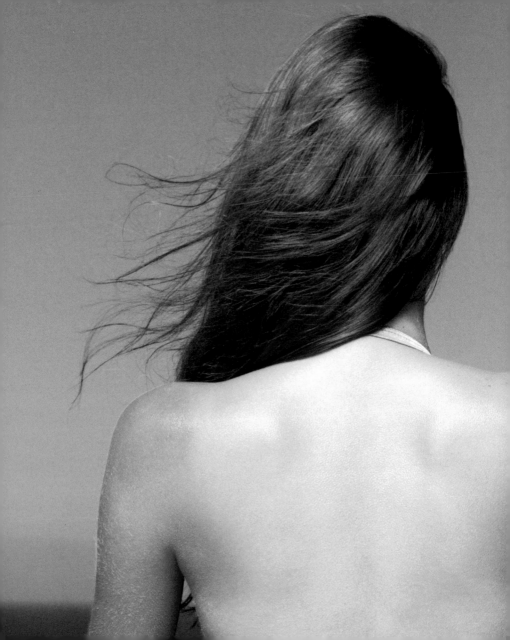

sunshine and your skin

Sunshine is made up of light from across a wide spectrum of wavelengths. It includes those wavelengths we can see – the visible spectrum – and those we can't, such as infra-red (heat) and ultra-violet (UV) radiation. Some sunlight is beneficial to health. It triggers production of vitamin D in the skin and helps prevent symptoms of Seasonal Affective Disorder (SAD), a form of depression linked to low levels of sunlight in the winter. But too much sunlight – especially from UV rays – can damage the skin. How much damage and what kind depends on the type of UV rays: UVA, UVB or UVC.

● ●

DID YOU KNOW? **MELANIN**

The skin' s main defence against sun damage is the brown pigment melanin, a natural filter against UV light. Melanin is produced in the lower layers of the skin and gradually migrates up towards the outer layers. Eventually, it reaches the surface and is lost along with the dead skin cells. Some manufacturers include ingredients in sun care products that are designed to increase production of melanin.

● ●

uv radiation

UVC radiation is absorbed by the earth's atmosphere and does not affect us, but UVB and UVA do reach us. UVB causes visible redness and burning (think 'B for Burning'). It does not penetrate the outer layer of skin, and so inflicts mainly short-term damage unless the burn is severe.

It is UVA that can cause serious, long-term damage. It penetrates deep into the skin where it brings about changes in living cells leading to premature ageing effects (think 'A for Ageing'). These changes are thought to be a primary cause of skin cancer.

sun filters and spfs

Sun lotions rely on filters to protect the skin from the damaging effects of UV radiation. The two categories of filter are physical filters and chemical filters.

physical filters

Physical filters act as a total barrier to UV radiation. Incorporated into a cream or lotion, these mineral filters form an invisible shield to prevent UV light from reaching the lower, living cells in the skin. Examples include the minerals titanium dioxide and zinc oxide. Once applied, physical filters keep working until they're wiped, washed or sweated off.

One potential drawback of physical filters is that they can make the skin appear blue-white. To avoid this problem, these minerals are very finely powdered, which reduces their capacity to reflect visible light, while still enabling them to reflect UV light.

chemical filters

Chemical filters convert UV light into less harmful forms of radiation, such as infra-red (heat). To do this, the chemical filter must change its structure, losing its sun-screen properties in the process – in other words it gets used up. For this reason, it is important to apply chemical filter-based lotions 30 minutes to one hour before sun exposure and reapply frequently.

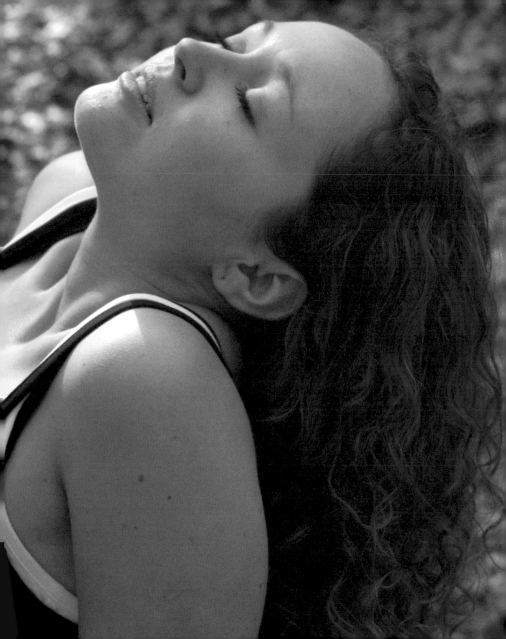

● ● ● ● ● ● ● ● ● ● ● ● ● ● ● ● ● ● ● ●

DID YOU KNOW? **OCTYL METHOXYCINNAMATE**

A common example of a chemical filter is octyl methoxycinnamate. Some
reports suggest this chemical may mimic hormones in the body, with
consequent potential health risks, especially to children and other susceptible
individuals. Another chemical sun filter, isoamyl p-methoxycinnamate, is
equally effective but does not have any hormone-like activity and so is
regarded as a safer alternative.

● ● ● ● ● ● ● ● ● ● ● ● ● ● ● ● ● ● ● ●

sun protection factors (spfs)

All products containing sun screens have a Sun Protection Factor
(SPF) number printed on them. The SPF indicates the level of
protection the product offers against UVB rays, which cause
visible burning. For example, SPF 8 will enable you to stay in the
sun for eight times as long as you could with no sun protection.
So, if your unprotected skin starts to burn after 15 minutes of sun
exposure, an SPF 8 product allows up to two hours exposure
before the skin starts to visibly burn. Similarly, an SPF 15 lotion
would allow almost four hours exposure to the same sunlight
before burning starts. However, this is no guide to the protection
the SPF offers against far more damaging UVA radiation.

SPF figures should not be taken too literally. For example,
SPF 30 does not give you twice as much protection as SPF 15.

When applied properly, sun lotion with SPF 30 protects you against 97 per cent of the UVB rays, while SPF 15 protects you against 93 per cent of UVB rays. In reality, the level of additional protection offered by SPF ratings higher than 25 is insignificant. Even at SPF 25, only 4 per cent of the UVB rays reach the skin. SPF ratings higher than 30 are primarily used as a marketing tool, and take advantage of the public's misconception of what protection ratings mean.

the star rating system

The Star Rating System was originally developed in Australia and is now owned by the Boots pharmaceutical company and used on its own-brand sun products and other proprietary brands. It consists of five levels of UVA protection, with one star indicating the lowest level and five stars the highest level.

To interpret the level of UVA protection a product offers correctly, you need to look at the star rating in conjunction with the SPF figure. For example, a product with a five-star rating and an SPF of 15 will offer greater UVA protection than a five-star product with an SPF of 8. Taken on its own, however, the star rating can be misleading. For example, a five-star SPF 8 lotion offers less UVA protection than a three-star SPF 15 lotion.

Without specialised knowledge, it is practically impossible to assess the UVA protection of a product using the star rating system alone and for this reason it has been largely dismissed by many scientists.

sun-protection tips

The most important step you can take to protect your skin from the sun is to use a sun lotion with the correct sun protection factor (SPF) for your skin type. Make sure that you apply it liberally and re-apply it frequently – especially after swimming or excessive sweating. You'll need to use a higher SPF factor for the first two days of sun exposure. In addition:

* Avoid the sun when it is strongest (11am – 3pm). Just 10 minutes unprotected exposure at this time can damage fair skin.
* If you're fair skinned, protect your skin even in the shade – 40 per cent of UV radiation can still reach you.
* Always keep babies out of direct sunlight on sunny days.
* Protect fair-skinned children with wide-brimmed hats and close-weave T-shirts and don't let children play in the water for too long without protection.
* Replace sun lotion annually – non-mineral UV-filters lose their efficacy over time, especially once the product has been opened.
* Protect your eyes from UV radiation, too (see page 139).

diet for uv protection

The most damaging effect of UV rays is to cause the production of free-radicals in the skin cells. Antioxidants, found in a wide variety of foods, can help protect the skin against free radicals. The best-known antioxidant is beta-carotene, found in leafy dark green vegetables and carrots. Lutein and zeaxanthin are found in dark green vegetables such as spinach, broccoli, green beans, green peas and kale.

Green tea contains a polyphenol called catechin, which has powerful protective properties. Drinking four cups of green tea a day will supply adequate protection against free radicals.

Other protective antioxidants are found in brightly coloured fruits and vegetables such as red, green and yellow peppers and dark berries such as bilberries, cherries and blackcurrants. To preserve antioxidants in vegetables, eat them raw or steam them. If you boil vegetables, don't discard the cooking water but leave it to cool and enjoy it as a refreshing drink, or use it as the basis for soups or stocks.

treating sunburn

Try the following natural treatments to ease discomfort and speed recovery of sunburn.

* Run a tepid bath, add a cupful of apple cider vinegar, a tablespoon of almond oil and 15 drops of lavender essential oil and mix well. The cider vinegar eases the sting, almond oil guards against dryness and lavender helps repair sun damage. This mixture also helps red skin turn brown without peeling.
* For small areas of sunburn, apply neat lavender essential oil.
* Aloe vera gel is soothing and cooling when applied to larger areas of sunburn. Add a few drops of peppermint oil to enhance aloe vera's cooling effect.

self tanning

Until recently, options for those who wanted a quick sun tan or a year-round tan were limited to fake tanning agents, such as bronzers, and solaria or sun beds/lamps. Now, new products are available, such as tanning accelerators and – currently the most popular – sunless tanners (see opposite).

bronzers

These colour the skin with a dye and, when applied professionally, can look convincing. They only last a few days, however, and so are best reserved for special occasions. Some bronzing dyes are synthetic, which may deter many people.

"Most solaria emit both UVB and UVA rays, responsible for wrinkling and ageing of the skin, as well as sunburn and skin cancer."

solaria

Sun beds and sun lamps expose the skin to the same forms of radiation as natural sunlight, and so the tan is the same as you get from sunbathing. But many experts believe the risks are the same too, so those wishing to avoid the dangers associated with sun exposure should treat sunbeds and sunray lamps with caution.

tanning accelerators

These encourage the body to produce the natural tanning pigment, melanin, more quickly. They do this by providing some of the building blocks or raw materials from which melanin is made, such as the amino acid tyrosine or the B vitamin inositol, extracted from the fruits of the carob tree.

These can increase tan density by almost 30 per cent over a two week period and so help you achieve a suntan with less exposure to damaging sunlight. They also increase the body's own natural defence against UV light. However, while these are perfectly safe to use, they do require some sun exposure to stimulate melanin production and so are not suitable for people who wish to avoid all exposure to sunlight.

sunless tanners

Sunless tanning products contain a colourless sugar called dihydroxyacetone (DHA). This reacts with amino acids in the surface skin cells to produce 'melanoidin', a substance chemically similar to the natural skin pigment melanin, causing skin coloration similar to a sun tan. DHA only affects the outermost dead cells of the epidermis and so does not damage the skin. It does not require exposure to UV light to work and so carries less risk than tanning accelerators.

The result depends on the formulation used, the user's complexion, and how it is applied (see tips). A colour change is usually apparent within a couple of hours of application but maximum darkening can take 8–24 hours to develop. If you want a darker colour, you may need to apply several successive applications every few hours. The tan lasts until the dead skin cells rub off, up to seven days with a single application. The same colour may be maintained with repeat applications every two to three days, depending on area.

As well as cosmetic uses, sunless tanning can be used clinically to treat vitiligo, a condition causing uneven skin pigmentation, or to camouflage skin irregularities, such as leg spider veins, or for individuals with photosensitivity disorders.

sunless tanning tips

You need care, skill and experience to get a good result from sunless tanning products. These tips can help you achieve a smooth and even look:

* Prepare the skin with thorough cleansing, then exfoliate using a sugar scrub, loofah or dry brushing to avoid uneven colour application. Take care when exfoliating your face – use a facial micro-fibre cloth or a gentle facial scrub.
* Wipe the skin with an acidic toner (such as a little vinegar in water) to remove any alkaline residues from soaps or detergents that may interfere with the tanner.

- ❋ Moisturise well, especially bony areas such as elbows, ankles, heels and knees.
- ❋ Apply sunless tanning lotion to your skin in thin layers wherever you want colour, using less on thicker skin, as colour stays longer in these areas.
- ❋ To avoid uneven darkening, use a wet cotton pad or damp flannel to remove excess cream from bony areas such as the elbows, ankles, heels and knees.
- ❋ To avoid tanned palms, use gloves when applying or wash your hands immediately afterwards.
- ❋ After applying sunless tanning lotion, wait 20–30 minutes for it to dry before you get dressed.
- ❋ Avoid shaving, showering, or swimming for at least an hour after application.
- ❋ Reapply regularly to maintain the colour.

DID YOU KNOW? **SUNLESS TANNERS**

Despite darkening of the skin after using sunless tanning lotion, you are still susceptible to harmful UV rays and so sun protection is still essential. Contact dermatitis due to DHA has been reported but is rare – most cases of sensitivity are due to other ingredients used in the cream or lotion base.

useful information

Where to Buy

All recommended supplements, digestive enzymes, psyllium husk, ground flax seeds, Omega blends, Scandinavian crisp bread, Yogi teas, fresh herbal juices and barley grass can be purchased from good health stores. Epsom salts can be obtained from most pharmacies. Organic, natural personal care products are available from www.greenpeople.co.uk. Other products mentioned in the text can be obtained from the following companies:

PAGE 19, mini trampoline
www.wholisticresearch.co.uk
PAGES 24 and 102, water
purifiers and filters
www.freshwaterfilter.com
www.ukjuicers.com
PAGE 37, pH Stix
www.healthleadsuk.com
PAGE 43, Hawthorn &
Artichoke Formula
www.greenpeople.co.uk
PAGE 189, Orgasmatron head
massager
www.whatwomenwant.co.uk

Addresses and Resources

Action Against Allergy
PO Box 278
Twickenham TW1 4QQ
020 8892 2711
www.actionagainstallergy.co.uk
email: AAA@actionagainst
allergy.freeserve.co.uk

British Association for
Nutritional Therapy
27 Old Gloucester Street
London WC1N 3XX
08706 061284
www.bant.org.uk
email: theadministrator@
bant.org.uk

British Society for Allergy
and Environmental Medicine
PO Box 7
Knighton
Powys LD7 2WF
01547 550380
www.jnem.demon.co.uk

The Cancer Prevention and
Education Society
10 Upper Bank Street
Canary Wharf
London E14 5JJ
www.cancerprevention
society.org
email: info@cancer
preventionsociety.org

Cancer Prevention Coalition
www.preventcancer.com

Foresight (the association for
pre-conceptual care)
28 The Paddock
Godalming
Surrey GU7 1KD
01483 427839
www.surreyweb.net

The Hale Clinic (centre for
complementary medicine)
7 Park Crescent
London W1B 1PF
020 7631 0156
www.haleclinic.com
email: admin@haleclinic.com

Health Kinesiology UK
44 Woodland Way
Old Tupton
Derbyshire S42 6JA
0870 765 5980
www.hk4health.co.uk/
register.htm

The Inside Story
Berrydales Publishers
Berrydale House
5 Lawn Road
London NW3 2XL
020 7722 2866
www.foodsmatter.com
email: info@insidestory.com

Kinesiology Federation
PO Box 28908
Dalkeith EH22 2YQ
0845 260 1094
www.kinesiologyfederation.org
email: kfadmin@kinesiology
federation.org

National Register of
Reflexologists
Dalton House
60 Windsor Avenue
London SW19 2RR
0800 0370130
www.reflexologyforum.org

Nutri People
483 Green Lanes
London N13 4BS
08701 999 332
www.nutripeople.co.uk

Organic Farmers and
Growers
Elim Centre
Lancaster Road
Shrewsbury
Shropshire SY1 3LE
0845 330 5122
www.organicfarmers.org.uk
email: info@organicfarmers.
org.uk

The Organic Food
Federation
31 Turbine Way
EcoTech Business Park
Swaffham
Norfolk PE37 7XD
01760 720444
www.orgfoodfed.com
email: info@orgfoodfed.com

Soil Association
South Plaza
Marlborough Street
Bristol BS1 3NX
0117 314 5000
www.soilassociation.org
e-mail: info@soilassociation.
org

The Vegan Society
Donald Watson House
21 Hylton Street
Hockley
Birmingham B18 6HJ
0121 523 1730
www.vegansociety.com

What Doctors Don't Tell You
Satellite House
2 Salisbury Road
London SW19 4EZ
0870 444 9886
www.wddty.com
e-mail: info@wddty.co.uk

Women's Environmental
Network
PO Box 30626
London E1 1TZ
020 7481 9004
www.wen.org.uk
email: info@wen.org.uk

The Wren Clinic
Centre for Natural Health
and Counselling
Idol Lane
London EC3R 5DD
020 7283 8908
www.wrenclinic.co.uk
email: info@wrenclinic.co.uk

YORKTEST Laboratories
Limited
G3, York Science Park
York YO10 5DQ
01904 410 410
www.allergy.co.uk
email: clientsupport@
yorktest.com

index

bibliography

Books

Baker, Sidney MacDonald *Detoxification and Healing* (McGraw-Hill Contemporary, 2003)

Caplin, Carole *LifeSmart* (Weidenfeld & Nicolson, 2004)

Clark, Susan *What Really Works* (HarperCollins, 2003)

Courteney, Hazel *500 of the Most Important Health Tips You'll Ever Need* (CICO Books, 2006)

— and Kathryn Marsden *Body Beauty Foods* (Reader's Digest, 1998)

Erasmus, Udo *Fats That Heal, Fats That Kill* (Alive Books, 1998)

Goodman, Jonathan *The Omega Solution* (Prima Lifestyles, 2001)

Grace, Janey Lee *Imperfectly Natural Woman* (Crown House, 2005)

Harper, Jennifer *Detox* (Dorling Kindersley, 2002)

— *9 Ways to Body Wisdom* (HarperCollins, 2000)

Holford, Patrick *Patrick Holford's New Optimum Nutrition Bible* (Piatkus Books, 2004)

— and Natalie Savona *Solve Your Skin Problems* (Piatkus Books, 2001)

Kenton, Leslie and Susannah *Authentic Woman* (Vermilion, 2005)

Lansky, Vicki *Vinegar* (Book Peddlers, 2004)

Marsden, Kathryn *The Complete Book of Food Combining* (Piatkus Books, 2005)

— *Good Gut Healing* (Piatkus Books, 2003)

— *Superskin* (HarperCollins, 2002)

McGuiness, Helen *Indian Head Massage* (Hodder Arnold, 2004)

McTaggart, Lynne *The Allergy Handbook* (What Doctors Don't Tell You, 1998)

Mehta, Narendra and Kundan, *The Face Lift Massage* (HarperCollins, 2004)

Morley, Carol, and Liz Wilde *Detox* (MQ Publications 2001)

Neal's Yard Remedies, *Recipes for Natural Beauty* (Haldane Mason, 2002)

Ryman, Daniele *Daniele Ryman's Aromatherapy Bible* (Piatkus Books, 2002)

Santillo, Humbart *Food Enzymes, The Missing Link to Radiant Health* (Hohm Press, U.S., 1993)

Stacey, Sarah, and Josephine Fairley, *The 21st Century Beauty Bible* (Kyle Cathie, 2004)

Steinman, David, and Samuel S. Epstein *The Safe Shopper's Bible* (MacMillan, 1995)

van Straten, Michael *The Complete Superfoods Cookbook* (Mitchell Beazley, 2007)

Vyas, Bharti, and Claire Haggard *Beauty Wisdom* (HarperCollins, 1998)

Watson, Francesca *Aromatherapy Blends and Remedies* (HarperCollins, 1995)

Wilde, Liz *Ageless* (Ryland, Peters & Small, 2006)

Winter, Ruth *A Consumer's Dictionary of Cosmetic Ingredients* (Three Rivers Press, 2005)

— *A Consumer's Dictionary of Food Additives* (Three Rivers Press, 2004)

Websites

www.dermatology.about.com/cs/skinanatomy/
a/anatomy.htm

www.greenpeace.org.uk

www.meddean.luc.edu/lumen/meded/
MEDICINE/dermatology/skinlsn/skin.htm

www.skincarephysicians.com/agingskinnet/
BasicFacts.html

www.wen.org.uk

www.wwf.org.uk

Articles

Aslama, M.N., E. Philip Lanskyb and
J. Varania 'Pomegranate as a cosmeceutical
source', *Journal of Ethnopharmacology*,
Volume 103, Issue 3, 20 February 2006,
pages 311–18.

Iliev, Emil, N. Tsankov and V. Broshtilova,
'Omega-3, -6 fatty acids in the
improvement of psoriatic symptoms',
Seminars in Integrative Medicine, Volume 1,
Issue 4, December 2003, pages 211–14.

Morenoa, D.A., M. Carvajala, C. López-
Berenguera and C. García-Viguera
'Chemical and biological characterisation
of nutraceutical compounds of broccoli',
*Journal of Pharmaceutical and Biomedical
Analysis*, Volume 41, Issue 5, 28 August
2006, pages 1508–22.

Wolf, R., H. Matz and E. Orion 'Acne and
diet' *Clinics in Dermatology*, Volume 22,
Issue 5, pages 387–93.

acknowledgements

I never envisaged that writing a book about my passion for organic health and beauty could be such an immense task. Writing a book is like entering a relationship with an obsessive partner who demands constant attention.

Firstly, I want to thank Ebury Press, Random House, specifically publishing director Carey Smith, for giving me the opportunity to write this book – a wonderfully exciting challenge, a journey I thoroughly enjoyed.

My copy editor, Richard Emerson, managed to trim the manuscript and his insight helped ensure that the information is clear, concise and logically organized. I would also like to thank designer Isobel Gillan and everyone at Ebury Press who had a hand in this book, particularly Clare Lawler, who had the initial idea about approaching Green People. Project editor Anne McDowall managed the project superbly and was always available to answer every one of my numerous questions promptly and completely.

I am deeply indebted to my colleagues Sue and Ian at Green People for their painstaking and thorough criticisms of this book. An extra big thank you to Ian for the many hours of proofreading, making sure that all of my sentences made sense. Thanks, too, to Jennifer for her heartwarming support.

Above all, I would like to give my special thanks to my partner Sven Erik who made my 'Green People' journey possible, and also a big thank you to our daughter Sandra whose patient love enabled me to complete this book.

CHARLOTTE VØHTZ

"Nobody grows old merely by living a number of years. We grow old by deserting our ideals. Years may wrinkle the skin, but to give up enthusiasm wrinkles the soul."

SAMUEL ULMANN